The Ketogenic Diet and Intermittent Fasting Secrets

Complete Beginner's Guide to the Keto Fast and Low-Carb Clarity Lifestyle; Discover Personalized Meal Plan to Reset your Life Today

Christine Moore

Contents

Powerful Ketogenic Diet and Intermittent Fasting Secrets _____ 1

Introduction _____ 3

Chapter 1:
Fundamentals of the Ketogenic Diet _____ 5

Chapter 2:
Ketosis _____ 28

Chapter 3:
Keto Nutritional Break Down _____ 36

Chapter 4:
Keto Meats and Nuts Products _____ 42

Chapter 5:
Keto Vegetable Products _____ 50

Chapter 6:
Keto Fruits, Dairy, and Oil Products _____ 55

Chapter 7:
Well Formulated Ketogenic Meals _____ 59

Chapter 8:
Finding Your Carb Sweet Spot _____ 62

Chapter 9:
Intermittent Fasting _____ 64

Chapter 10:
Why Try Intermittent Fasting _____ 77

Chapter 11:
Keto and Intermittent Fasting _____ 88

Chapter 12:
Intermittent Fasting Regiments _____ 93

Chapter 13:
Beginners 4 Week Plan _____ 99

Chapter 14:
Big No No's _____ 119

Chapter 15:
Tips and Tricks and FAQs _____ 123

Conclusion _____ 142

Anti-Inflammatory Keto (30% More Effective) _____ 143

Introduction _____ 145

Chapter 1:
The Ketogenic Diet_____ 148

Chapter 2:
Ketosis _____ 155

Chapter 3:
The Nutritional Break Down _____ 163

Chapter 4:
Dirty Keto _____ 167

Chapter 5:
The Mediterranean Diet _____ 175

Chapter 6:
Ketogenic Mediterranean Diet _____ 186

Chapter 7:
Keto-Mediterranean Vegetables _____ 195

Chapter 8:
Keto Mediterranean Meats and Nuts_____ 200

Chapter 9:
Keto-Mediterranean Fruits and Dairy Products ____ 211

Chapter 10:
Finding Your Carb Sweet Spot_____ 220

Chapter 11:
Intermittent Fasting _____ 234

Chapter 12:
The Mediterranean Ketogenic Diet _____ 244

Chapter 13:
Foods to Eat on IF and Sample Meal Plan _____ 248

Chapter 14:
Fourteen: Common Mistakes _____ 254

Chapter 15:
Tips and Tricks _____ 260

Chapter 16:
Frequently Asked Questions _____ 272

Conclusion _____ 285

THE KETOGENIC DIET

AND

INTERMITTENT FASTING

Secrets

COMPLETE BEGINNER'S GUIDE TO THE KETO FAST AND
LOW-CARB CLARITY LIFESTYLE: DISCOVER PERSONALIZED
MEAL PLAN TO RESET YOUR LIFE TODAY

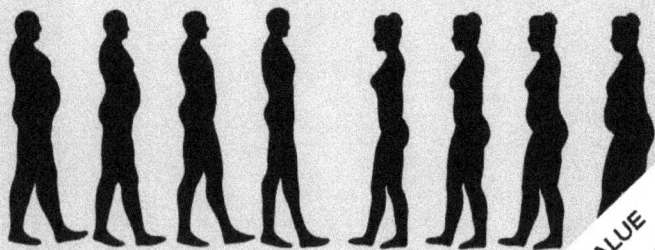

CHRISTINE MOORE

2 IN 1 VALUE

Powerful Ketogenic Diet and Intermittent Fasting Secrets

Complete Keto Fast Guide to Gain the Low-Carb Clarity Lifestyle in 21 Days
and Burn Fat - Includes Autophagy, OMAD, Meal Plan Content

Christine Moore

POWERFUL

Ketogenic

DIET

AND

INTERMITTENT
FASTING

Secrets

COMPLETE KETO FAST GUIDE TO GAIN THE LOW-CARB
CLARITY LIFESTYLE IN 21 DAYS AND BURN FAT - INCLUDES
AUTOPHAGY, OMAD, MEAL PLAN CONTENT

CHRISTINE MOORE

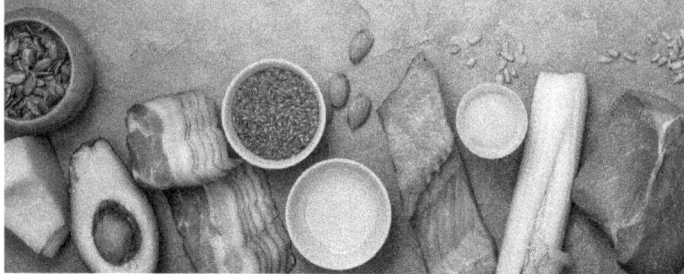

Introduction

Beginning a new lifestyle can be daunting. It doesn't matter even if you know that the lifestyle promises many benefits such as weight loss and improved health without the drawbacks of crash or fad diets. A lifestyle change will impact your life, and you can be unsure on how to approach the change. But there is no need to fear. In this book, you will learn all you need to know about the Ketogenic diet, how to transition onto it fully within thirty days, manage any side effects, pair it with helpful exercises and intermittent fasting, and much more to get you well on your way toward success.

I have designed this book in a way that it is easy to understand the secrets of the Ketogenic diet, ketosis, and the countless health benefits associated with this lifestyle change alongside intermittent fasting. This whole book will help you shift to the Ketogenic world without any fears.

Ketogenic diets have been in use for thousands of years for their many health benefits, ease of implementation, and simply because of the environments we evolved in.

Even if you are a beginner to the diet, you will be able to adapt easily. Because this diet works to improve health while also decreasing weight, it has become a popular choice for everyone who wishes to lose weight, live a healthy lifestyle, or both. It is the best way to rapidly lose weight without sacrificing your health or taking harmful drugs.

The Ketogenic diet is very scientific in how it works. It is designed to put the body in a state of ketosis. You attain this state when your body starts burning fat stores for fuel, instead of sugars. As you can imagine, burning the storage of fat is exactly what you need to do to lose the type of weight that you want to lose, while maintaining your muscles.

Along with burning fat stores, ketosis has a neurological effect that will leave you feeling happier and less hungry. Both results will further help you lose any amount of weight you want. Because it is a healthy way to eat, you can continue with the Ketogenic diet indefinitely to maintain the ideal weight for your body type.

Chapter 1:
Fundamentals of the Ketogenic Diet

The word Ketogenic is getting a lot of hype these days and comes to the limelight more often than before. Since the whole diet plan of the book centers on a Ketogenic lifestyle, we will dive deeper to expand your understanding of the Ketogenic Diet.

Ketogenic diet refers to a group comprising many regimens that are known to contain low amounts of carbs with "high-fat, moderate protein" or "moderate fat, high-protein." The meaning of Keto originates from a metabolic process that occurs in the body called Ketosis. The process is essential in contributing toward the loss of that extra pound.

What is Ketosis? It is a healthy and natural metabolic process taking place in the body in which stored fat is burned to release some chemicals known as the Ketones. The ketones are essential in lowering fat levels in the human body and provide energy for various activities we undertake. When there is a scarcity of carbohydrate from the food you take, the fat in your body is burnt to provide that energy, which your carbs could not offer. Because of the process, production of ke-tones occurs. More will be explained later.

The Ketogenic diet involves high consumption of fats, a limited intake of proteins, and an almost limited intake of carbohydrates. The limited glucose intake can trigger satiety and allow you to attain a state of ketosis, which is the metabolism of fats for energy. This aids to has-ten a healthy weight loss process without having to resort to starva-tion. Many may find this concept unappealing and questionable as there exists public knowledge linking fats as a cause of heart dis-eases. Moreover, skeptics do not believe its claim of getting rid of fatty deposits in the body by eating more fats as it is essentially fighting fire with fire.

The Ketogenic diet has become a wildly popular diet in recent years. However, the Ketogenic diet is not new. In fact, it has been in practice since the 1920s when it was originally created as a treatment for ep-ilepsy. Also called "Keto," this diet focuses on changing eating habits to center on lower carb intake. The objective is to ensure that you ingest less than 50g of the net carbohydrates each day, not including carbs from fiber, so that the body can transition into a state of keto-sis.

It is intended to make sure the body gets enough protein and nutrients to stay healthy and energized, but not so many that it gains weight.

Over the years, as the diet gained popularity, it began to be used for additional therapies, including the treatment of rare metabolic diseases, brain tumors, autism, depression, migraine headaches, and even Type 2 Diabetes. It has also been in extensive use for traumatic brain injuries, strokes, Parkinson's, and Alzheimer's disease. Oncologists even recommend this diet to cancer patients.

Many people struggling with weight issues and health conditions are always on the lookout for diets that can work for them and grant the desired results. Finding diets that can provide sustained results over long-term has been a challenge. Ketogenic diet is good for losing weight and to maintain a healthy lifestyle in the long-term. For a diet plan to be effective; it shouldn't be just capable of yielding the desired results; it should also be one that many find to be enjoyable.

When you have been eating in each way for your entire life; finding instant changes when you start on a new diet such as the Ketogenic diet may not be automatic as the body takes time to completely shift and adapt to the new lifestyle. The human body was never designed to burn sugar for energy, going by human history. The craze about sugar is something that has been adopted recently however, even the ancestors lived their lives off meat and vegetables. The human bodies were designed to burn fat for fuel and the body has been proven to operate at optimum when utilizing fat for fuel.

Following a Ketogenic diet enables the body to burn fat for fuel which in turn accelerates weight loss alongside increased energy levels. Maintaining a healthy lifestyle is then possible without focusing much on restricting intake of calories, or even eating boring and bland meals to attain the desired results.

In a Ketogenic diet, you take high-fat and low-carb food for a longer period to start the process of ketosis in your body. You ingest protein in moderate. The reduction of carbohydrates in your body allows the already available fat to take its place.

When a person is on Ketogenic diet, the body gets to burn fat for fuel instead of burning sugar for fuel as it normally happens when one is on high carb diet. Being on this diet completely changes the functioning of the body but in quite a good way. It is based on the premise that the human body is designed to burn fat for energy instead of sugar.

When you consume foods that have high levels of carbs, the body gets to produce glucose and insulin. The body prefers use of glucose since the conversion of glucose molecule to energy is much easier. Insulin also gets produced to help with processing glucose to the blood-stream by transporting it all through the body. When glucose is uti-lized as the primary source of energy, the fats that gets consumed doesn't get utilized and instead ends up being stored in the body. Go-ing by an average person's diet; glucose is normally the main source of energy. It may not bring much problem for the body especially when one is involved in high energy activities that ensure most of the energy that gets consumed is utilized.

A problem arises when the body produces more glucose than what is required. The extra glucose then gets converted to fat which then gets stored. Since the body utilizes glucose as the main source of energy, the glucose that gets converted to fat is never used. Whenever the body runs out of glucose, the brain sends signals that you want more glucose, so you are more likely to feel cravings for sugary things or a piece of snack. Being in such a cycle leads to development of a body that's not only overweight but also prone to several health-related diseases.

The process of carb reduction enhances the efficiency of your metabolic state known as ketosis. The fat starts burning faster and turns into ketones. These ketones provide more energy to enhance your mental power. Similarly, this diet also reduces the insulin and blood sugar content in your body. All in all, your body obtains multiple health benefits with a disciplined diet of Ketogenic.

Despite its benefits, the Ketogenic diet isn't for everybody. It requires strict tracking of your intake at the beginning to ensure that you're staying under the maximum of carbohydrates allowed (50 grams), which can be a deterrent to some. It's also not an easy diet to follow as it almost completely cuts off access to the comfort foods and cravings that we typically reach for. Basically, anything with refined sugar in it is a big "no."

Types of Keto

Standard Ketogenic Diet (SKD) – It is the type of Keto that has high-fats, low carbs and moderate protein each day. Standard percentages include 5% of carbs, 75% of fat, and about 20% of protein. The objective of the diet is to ensure that the body enters the state of ketosis to enable weight loss and decrease the frequency of epileptic seizures.

The diet does not allow the consumption of fruits, starches and milk. People feed on cheese, oils, butter and fatty meats. The diet allows carbs of under 30 grams. It is not advisable to work out when following the diet since there is not much energy due to fewer carbs ingested.

SKD is not good for individuals who work out regularly. It is good for sedentary people, obese people and those who are not willing to exercise. The diet is known to regulate hunger, controls intake of carbs and triggers fat loss process without the need of working out. You need to strictly follow for seven days consecutively.

When one consumes a low number of calories for a longer period, it may slow down metabolism which may prevent further weight loss. In the absence of occasional high carb in a diet, Ghrelin and Leptin (which are fat loss hormones) cannot be reset. You are advised not to stay on a diet for long.

After successful weight loss and you can work out, you can switch to the other Keto types which have more carbs that allow for more activity and will reset the Leptin and Ghrelin.

Targeted Ketogenic Diet (TKD) – The diet allows you to have an intake of carbs that range between 25 and 50 grams when you must work out. The carbs should be enough to sustain exercising without influencing ketosis. You have the option of working out three times a week. The targeted type of Ketogenic diet is decided by the workout you include. You can increase or decrease the carbohydrate content in your food depending on your workout's intensity.

Cyclical Ketogenic Diet (CKD) – The diet requires you to adhere to a strict version for five days and to binge on carbs for the remaining two days. Hence, the body smoothly converts the body fat into energy. It is easier to adhere to this type of diet since it allows you to have as many carbs as possible during the two days.

High Protein Ketogenic Diet: This one resembles the diet patterns of the standard type. However, you take about 35% of protein when following this Ketogenic diet. The fat portion stays 60%, while the carbs included are 5% only. Sports personalities, athletes, and bodybuilders utilize targeted and cyclical methods popularly.

History of Keto

Keto diet is a technique developed by modern physicians in the 1920's for treatment of epilepsy. The Keto diet is a high-fat diet with a moderate level of protein and low in carbohydrate in medicine used to treat epilepsy in children. The Ketogenic diet makes the human body to begin burning fats instead of carbohydrates. Keto diet therapy was developed as an alternative option for nonmainstream fasting. Doctors noticed that some epilepsy patients have exhibited signs of starving and some patients have low blood sugar. For many years, mankind new that fasting was geared towards the treatment of several diseases. This was studied in detail by ancient Indian physicians and ancient Greek physicians. An early discourse in the Hippocratic Corpus, "On the Sacred Disease," gives details how diet changes helped in management of epilepsy. In 1911, the first scientific study of fasting was used as a treatment for epilepsy in France. The experiment was conducted on twenty epileptic patients; all were detoxed by consuming a low-calorie vegetarian diet.

Advantages of Keto

Many people have claimed how being on Ketogenic diet changed their life and that's a fact that has been proven by many. Ketogenic diet is much more than a diet, it's a lifestyle that provides numerous benefits.

Weight Loss: One of the major motivations of being on Ketogenic diet is for weight loss. When on Ketogenic diet, the body uses fat as a source of energy and will then begin burning the unwanted fat which eventually leads to weight loss. Since the body can't take energy from carbs and sugars, the ketosis directs the system to draw energy from stored fat deposits and as you have guessed it, it gets this energy by burning these fat cells first. When on Keto diet, the level of fat storing hormone insulin drops, which then allows the fat cells to travel to the liver where it gets converted to ketones. The body eventually becomes a fat burning machine which makes weight loss to be much easier. Other than the ketosis process, a Keto diet can help you lose weight because of several reasons.

First, as opposed to processed snacks and other high carbohydrate foods, eating fat makes you eat less due to the effective satiating effect it induces on your metabolism. When you eat foods like cheese, fatty fish, avocado and nuts, the fat content gets into the intestines and triggers release of hormones. Such hormones among them are the cholecystokinin and Peptide YY to help control satiety and appetite and can make you feel fuller for longer. The satiating effect of fat is linked to its complexity in chemical composition that demands for a longer time to digest and extra energy to break down. A scientific study found out polyunsaturated fats, commonly referred to as "PUFAs," can trigger fullness to a bigger extent than meals with lower fatty acids. Eating a high-fat diet can also help you stick to your diet plan and in turn burn extra fat or lose weight.

Secondly, fat speeds up the rate of metabolism compared to a low-fat or high carb diet due to its link with fat burning hormones called adipokines. Hormones such as adiponectin are formed from fat cells and their work is to boost the rate at which fats are metabolized. To further explain the importance of eating fats, a study found out that eating healthier fat can help speed up metabolism and reduce storage of visceral or belly fat. Findings in this study showed that people who consumed high-fat foods burned 300 more calories daily compared to the low-fat group. Better still, the high-fat group had a normal amount of blood insulin and was less likely to develop related diabetic conditions. The high-fat group fed on 60 percent fats, 30 percent proteins and only 10 percent carbs while the low-fat group consumed 60 percent carbs, 20 percent fats and 20 percent proteins.

In addition, fat acts as a solvent for fat-soluble nutrients such as vitamin A, D, E, and K. The body needs to absorb such nutrients to facilitate various metabolic functions, and deficiency of these nutrients can be detrimental. Insufficient amounts of vital minerals and vitamins may result in problems such as blood clots, blindness, brittle bones among others. For weight loss, you need vitamin D, as it helps metabolize body fat from regions such as the abdomen.

Controls Blood Sugar: when one is on a high carbohydrate diet; the body reaches a state where it's unable to handle the higher levels of insulin in the body. A person is then more likely to develop medical conditions such diabetes and increased blood sugar levels. When a person switches to a low carb diet, the blood sugar levels gets lowered which makes Ketogenic diet suitable for those with diabetes type 2. The diet also enables people to maintain consistent levels of blood sugar and overall improvement of health.

Mental Focus: it's not easy to understand how being on a high carb diet leads to having a cloudy way of thinking until you are off the diet. Mental focus is one of the major benefits that come with being on a Ketogenic diet. The diet that you are on has a substantial effect on your state of mental health as the brain requires almost 25% of the calories consumed to be able to execute various activities. The increased fat intake when you are on a Ketogenic diet helps in improving the functioning of the brain in various ways. Being on a diet that's not balanced leads to lack of mental clarity and that is likely to show up as having difficulty in remembering things, feelings of a foggy brain and inability to stay focused.

Ketones provide the body with a source of energy that enables it to process efficiently the extra glutamate into GABA and eventually decreases then reduces stimulation and improved mental focus. Most of the brain tissue consists of fatty acids so being on a high-fat diet leads to improved mental focus. The essential fatty acids such as omega-6 and omega-3 are very crucial for brain health. Being on Ketogenic diet also improves one's memory. Being on ketosis state helps in production of mitochondria and eventually increases the brain's memory cells.

Increased Levels of Energy: Being on Ketogenic diet brings to end feelings of fatigue naturally. You will then realize that you have a clearer mind with better moods. Most of the high carb and traditional diets are centered around foods that are sugary and have starchy carbs. These carbs normally spike and increase levels of insulin in the body which eventually results into high blood sugar levels. A rapid rise in levels of insulin also causes sluggishness and increased feelings of lethargy.

Once a person shifts to a low carb, high-fat diet, they also get to experience increased levels of energy, less compulsive eating and cravings for carbs, and better mental concentration. With increased feelings of alertness and less need for sleep also come increased levels of energy.

Reduce Triglycerides: Triglycerides are a certain type of fat present in the blood. Once food is consumed, the body converts the food into glucose with the excess calories being converted into triglycerides for storage in the body cells. Being on a high carb diet increases the level of triglycerides which then gets reduced when one shifts to low carb diet. Reduced levels also lower chances of contracting ailments.

Reduced Cholesterol: consumption of high carb foods has the potential of increasing levels of cholesterol in the body with great chances of causing heart disease or stroke. There is the high-density lipoprotein (HDL) which is also known as the good cholesterol and the low-density lipoprotein (LDL) also referred to as the bad cholesterol. LDL is known to transport cholesterol present in the liver and other body parts which then creates a buildup around the arteries. HDL is involved in the carrying of cholesterol from other parts of the body to the liver where they get utilized or excreted out of the body. Being on Ketogenic diet reduces the level of bad cholesterol which then re-sults into reduced risks of heart disease and other ailments.

Treatment for Metabolic Syndrome: this is a medical condition that's associated with the risk of heart disease and diabetes. The con-dition consists of a collection of symptoms such as the ones below;

- Abdominal obesity

- High triglycerides

- Low HDL levels

- High levels of blood sugar

- Elevated blood pressure

Improved Digestion: Improved digestion depends on the health of the gut as over 70% of the immune system is found in the gut. A high carb diet tends to release sugar, antibiotics, additives, and pesticides that affect the good bacteria required along the intestinal tract for efficient digestion. A shift to Ketogenic diet enables the body to burn fat for fuel which results into production of more good bacteria while eliminating the bad bacteria. The result is an improved digestive system.

Treating Gastrointestinal Problems: digestive issues like irritable bowel syndrome, acid reflux, gallstones, inflammation, bloating, heartburn can lead to chronic diseases if not controlled. A change in your diet can fix all this. Keto diet helps in improving your eating habits and reduces the discomfort caused due to an irritable gut.

Epilepsy Control: The Keto diet has been utilized for nearly a century to help treat patients suffering from seizures and Epilepsy. Even to this day, it is widely used by major health clinics e.g. Mayo Clinic to treat kids and young adults suffering from the disease. While it can't cure Epilepsy (which has no cure to this day), it can certainly help control the number of medications needed to control Epilepsy symptoms and ease inflammation of the nervous system.

Acne and Eczema: another health benefit of the Keto diet, which not many people are aware of, is helping ease acne and eczema breakouts, as well as other inflammatory skin disorders (dermatitis, scalp issues). The Keto diet can do this by decreasing inflammation inside the body and encouraging tissue cells to repair themselves faster and more effectively than before. It appears to have the opposite effect of following high-carb and high-sugar diets, which have been found to indirectly cause acne and skin inflammation in general.

Reduced Risk of Heart Disease: A Ketogenic diet helps in regulating the levels of blood sugar and lowers the blood pressure levels. Since it is a low-carb and high-fat diet, it leads to a reduction of triglycerides and cholesterol. This is because of the increase in the levels of HDL (good cholesterol) while reducing the levels of LDL (bad cholesterol). A high level of HDL indicates a lower risk of cardiac diseases.

Improves Women's Health: A Keto diet helps in strengthening fertility. Polycystic Ovarian Syndrome is a widespread hormonal disorder in women, and it can be treated and controlled by following the Keto diet. This diet also helps in overcoming other symptoms like acne and obesity. It regularizes the menstrual cycle as well.

Strengthens the Eyes: increased amounts of sugar in an individual's system can be toxic and can deteriorate eyesight. This increases the risk of cataracts, and a diet that drastically cuts down on sugar reduces such risks as well.

Controls Appetite: hunger pangs can make many individuals give up on a certain diet. A Keto diet is rich in fats, and this makes you feel fuller for longer, in a healthy way. Unintentionally, your calorie intake reduces too.

Dangers of the Ketogenic Diet

Keto diet is a safe diet plan, but it may lead to some side effects. I think I should let you know that there are some changes which you might face during the early days of your Keto diet due to changes in your body's overall homeostatic functions.

There are a few different side-effects of the Ketogenic diet that you should be aware of. Some of them might be uncomfortable or annoying at first, but they are temporary. You just need to stick with the diet for a week or so before you see some improvement.

However, these symptoms will eventually go away! So, don't be alarmed if you face any of such symptoms like aggravation, Keto-Flu and Mental Fogginess among other explained below.

Physical Performance: one the main side effects of the Ketogenic diet is a temporary lull in physical performance. You might see some limitations when you first begin this diet, but as the body adapts and adjusts to using fat as its primary source of fuel, all your endurance and strength will return.

Effect on Liver, Muscles and Frequent Urination: carbohydrate is stored in our bodies mainly in the liver and muscles in the form of glycogen. An individual requires approximately 600 calories to sustain daily without eating anything. But if you are not into too much of exercising and have been leading a sedentary life most of your life, the carbohydrate starts to accumulate. On the other hand, if you exercise rigorously and your carb intake is low, you will have exhausted the glycogen very soon. But at the same time, you experience fatigue and tend to get dehydrated, which is not good for your health. Since there is little carbohydrate left and you carry on with the normal daily activities, you gradually get dehydrated. So, if you are opting for Ketogenic diet, you ought to do away with rigorous exercise and intense weight training.

After the first day or two of the diet, you'll most likely notice that you're making some more frequent trips to the bathroom. Your body is burning up those extra glycogen stores in the liver and muscles. Breaking down the glycogen will release a lot of water. As your carbohydrate intake and your glycogen stores decrease, your kidneys are going to begin getting rid of this excess water.

In addition, as the levels of insulin circulating through your body lower, your kidneys will begin excreting some excess sodium, which is going to cause more frequent urination. This side effect will eventually cease.

Risk of Cancer: if you are on a low carbohydrate diet, and if you are not able to maintain it properly with the right number of elements, you will have trouble with digestion and lead to bowel and constipation irregularities. This makes you susceptible to cardiovascular diseases and digestive cancer. Also, another cause of concern is that if you deprive yourself of legume, fruits, vegetables, and grains, it results in insufficient intake of potassium, vitamin C, and antioxidants. Also, intake of phytonutrients is compromised.

Prone to Heart Disease: there are a few categories of high-fat food items that include egg yolks, coconut, and lard. These have a high saturated fat content but low carbohydrate as well as protein content. Consuming this kind of food over a long period of time makes you susceptible to heart diseases. Also, it has been observed that a diet high in fat content have a detrimental effect on the brain cells. This is because there is a set of brain cells that regulate body weight.

Dizziness and Fatigue: as you begin getting rid of water, you're going to lose some minerals such as potassium, salt, and magnesium. Lower levels of these minerals can cause lightheadedness, dizziness, and fatigue. It can also cause headaches, muscle cramps and skin itchiness.

To reduce these side effects, consume enough replacement minerals. Consume more sea salt and drink some salty broth. In addition, eat foods high in minerals, such as leafy green vegetables and avocados.

If your carbohydrate consumption is lower than sixty carbohydrates per day, you'll need to carry on eating a moderate amount of salt. However, if you are under high blood pressure medication, you need to check with a doctor first.

In addition, you might want to take a magnesium supplement of 400mg before bed every night. If you have heart or kidney conditions, check with a doctor before taking this dose.

It's also important to eat at least two cups of raw, green leafy vegetables each day. These provide you with vitamin K and potassium and will help greatly with hunger cravings.

Low Blood Sugar (Hypoglycemia): with a higher carbohydrate diet, the body releases insulin to convert carbs to glucose. When you abruptly decrease that carbohydrate intake on the Ketogenic diet plan, you might have some fleeting low blood sugar incidents.

Headaches: as your body adapts to the ketosis, headaches can come about for a few different reasons. You could feel lightheaded and feel like you have the flu for a few days. This is usually due to mineral deficiencies. To see if it's from sodium, try putting a quarter of a teaspoon of salt into a glass of water and drink it. You should feel better in about twenty minutes.

Increase your salt and water intake to reduce headache symptoms. These should improve after few days. If not, add a few more carbuhydrates to your daily total.

Constipation: usually the same cause as frequent urination, salt loss. Can also be caused by magnesium imbalances or excess nuts or dairy consumption. The intake of magnesium supplement of 400mg will help with this. If 400mg of magnesium citrate doesn't help, then you might want to cut back on how much dairy you consume in order to balance out your calcium intake. Drinks tons of water and monitor nut and dairy consumption.

Sugar Cravings: this is very common. People may laugh, but sugar cravings can be just as bad as any other addictive product. As your body goes through the process of burning fat rather than sugar, there is a two to twenty-one-day period where carbohydrate cravings can be quite intense. If you can wait it out, then the cravings will disappear. Be strong! Eating a huge amount of carbohydrates will bring those cravings right back, and halt ketosis. For some people, eating sugar in any amount starts the process all over again.

Diarrhea: this isn't an unusual side effect of a low carbohydrate diet, and it should resolve after a few days. This can result from eating too much protein and not enough fat. Eating a high protein, low carbohydrate, low-fat diet causes symptoms that are known as rabbit starvation. Be sure you replace the carbohydrates you cut out of your diet with more fat.

Weakness or Shakiness: this is one of the side effects of the hypoglycemia you can experience. It's also a symptom of low amounts of minerals in your system. Add a little more protein to your diet and eat more salt. In addition, include more foods with potassium. You can also take a 99mg potassium citrate supplement to help offset this symptom.

Muscle Cramps: this is another side effect of losing minerals, especially magnesium. Take three slow release magnesium tablets for twenty days, and then continue to take one tablet each day after twenty days.

Sleeping Problems: some individuals report difficulty sleeping while following the Keto Diet. This may indicate low serotonin or insulin levels. Try eating a snack that has protein and a little carbohydrate right before you go to bed. The carbohydrates release insulin, which lets more tryptophan from the protein you consumed get into the brain. This is a precursor to serotonin, which has an overall calming effect.

Sleep problems may also be caused by histamine intolerance. Low carbohydrates foods often contain high amounts of histamines, and some people will react to a higher intake of these types of foods with sleeplessness and anxiety.

Kidney Stones: some people bring this side effect up when they try to convince people that a low carbohydrate diet is dangerous. They base this on reports of calcium-based kidney stones reported by physicians who used the Ketogenic diet for children who had epilepsy. However, this is not a very accurate comparison.

First, the diet that is given to children with epilepsy contains close to 90% fat and processed powders that are used to make shakes used a lot for children who have epilepsy. A real Ketogenic food diet is different and includes more protein. However, if you're worried about it, a citrate supplement can minimize your risk.

Lowered T3 Thyroid Hormones: while this side effect is usually viewed as negative, it's a natural result of a ketosis lower calorie diet. The same thing happens on calorie-restricted high carbohydrate diets.

In addition, it's possible your body becomes more sensitive to the T3 when you're in ketosis state, as your body requires less of this hormone to get the job done.

Racing Heart or Heart Palpitations: some people experience heart palpitations when they begin a Keto diet or after they've been on one for a few weeks or months. It's been reported this is more likely to happen if the person has a low blood pressure normally. There are a few other potential factors that may cause heart palpitations.

Nutrient Deficiency - A multivitamin that has the RDA for selenium and zinc, as well as a magnesium supplement, is strongly recommended. You can also try some homemade bone broth.

Insulin Resistance - transient hypoglycemia can result from not eating often enough or not eating enough fat and protein.

Electrolyte imbalance or Dehydration - Making some mineral water at home and drinking a cup in the morning and one in the evening can help if this is your problem. In addition, be sure you consume plenty of water to avoid dehydration.

Too much MCT or Coconut Oil - As you add these to your diet, begin with small amounts and increase them over time. Never rely on coconut oil as your only fat intake. Be sure you include other fats, such as ghee, butter, animal fats, and olive oil, too.

Hair Loss: although rare, some people report experiencing accelerated hair loss while following the Keto diet. This is not related directly to the Ketogenic diet but is associated with a change in diet. This process is known as telogen effluvium, a medical term for hair loss due to a change in hormone levels or metabolism. Ketogenic diets create a lower insulin level, which is one of the main hormones in the human body, and hair loss can be a natural but temporary side effect.

Remember, these are potential side effects. You may experience these side effects, you may not! However, it is good to be prepared for what potential effects to expect. These side effects are temporary. Once your body adjusts to the diet, they should subside.

Chapter 2:
Ketosis

As the carbohydrate is reduced in the human body, it starts utilizing the available fat as fuel. The whole body starts to get energy from fat only. Ketosis is a metabolic state that gets induced when the body begins to use fats as the main source of fuel instead of carbohydrates. The body while in such a metabolic process gets to break down the stored fats as source of energy instead of glucose since the body is deprived of enough carbs that can be converted into glucose. The reason for being on Ketogenic diet is so that the body can get into a metabolic state which is referred to as ketosis. The event of ketosis occurs in your body during strict diet or fasting conditions.

In terms of health benefits, ketosis offers quick loss of weight, increased performance level of the body, and improved health condition of the heart. However, excessive ketosis can prove to be harmful to certain diabetic patients.

Ketogenic diet is an effective way to maximize the process of ketosis. Regular high-fat and low-carbohydrate diet helps in replacing the glucose with the ketone molecules. Hence, all the body fat burns simultaneously as you take them. As a result, your body starts losing weight, which you can control according to your weight goals.

Ketosis is principally dependent on the bodily levels of three essential components: glucagon, insulin and blood glucose. The entire process starts and ends with metabolism.

As mentioned above, the body breaks down ingested substances to use as fuel for the body; namely carbohydrates, fats, and proteins (in that order). When the primary source is about to run dry, the body moves on to the substance that is second in line and, when this too has a low supply, it uses the tertiary choice.

Under normal circumstances, blood glucose levels are kept within a healthy range by insulin. It does so by facilitating the transport of glucose from the bloodstream into body cells. If the pancreas fails to produce an adequate amount of insulin, there would be an unmanageable and potentially harmful level of glucose in the blood.

Glucagon, on the other hand, is considered as the "antagonistic hormone" of insulin. This substance, which is also secreted by the pancreas, is produced when insulin levels fall low. Such a situation emanates inadequate consumption of carbohydrates and meal-skipping. It works by turning the glycogen present in the liver into a simpler form - glucose. However, if this process goes on until there is a depletion of glycogen supply in the liver, the pancreas will begin to break down lipids (also known as fatty acids) into ketone bodies to use as energy. This secondary means of fueling the body is known as ketosis.

How Ketosis Works

When the level of glycogen and glucose are depleted in the body; the levels of insulin and blood sugar also gets to decrease, and the body is then forced to look for alternative energy source. The body then begins to break down the stored fats for energy through a process that's referred to as beta-oxidation, which leads to increased levels of acetoacetate. Acetoacetate then forms the ketone body that gets transported through the blood and to the brain for provision of energy.

When the body produces enough ketones with significant levels of over 0.5mM in the blood, it's already in ketosis state. One of the fastest ways of getting the body to ketosis is through fasting. When the body is deprived of food, it automatically switches to utilizing the stored fats for energy. When getting started on a Ketogenic diet, beginners can consider engaging in periods of fasting so that the body gets to switch to ketosis state much faster.

One of the common misconceptions associated with being on a high carb diet is that the brain needs carbs to be able to function effectively. The truth is that the brain happily burns ketones and intake of carbs may not be necessary at all. To attain the metabolic state of ketosis, foods should be consumed in the ratio of 75% or more of fats, 20% or less of proteins and 5% or less of carbohydrates. There are plenty of foods that you can choose from at every meal to be able to reach the required macronutrients ratios.

How do You Know You Are in Ketosis?

There are technical and general ways to find out and ensure that you are in ketosis. You can get your blood samples tested, or the same with urine samples as well as breath samples. Generally, there are visible signs that tell you that you have successfully achieved ketosis:

Increased Desire for Drinking Water: Dry mouth is a common sign that you are going through ketosis. The desire for drinking water increases due to that. This happens because your body asks for electrolytes. People using Ketogenic diet are recommended 2 cups of bouillon every day along with large quantities of water.

Fruity Smell: Incredible right? The production of ketones also creates acetone as the by-product in the cells. This acetone comes out when you exhale. Hence, the breath gives a fruity smell. It generally smells like a flavored nail polish. The similar smell is possible when you sweat, especially during an intense workout. However, the fruity breath stays only for a little while.

Increased Urge of Urination: During the initial period of Ketogenic diet, you can experience an increased urge for urination. The creation of ketones in your body also sends some acetoacetate to your urine. The consistent creation of ketones increases the level of urine generation as well. Hence, you end up in the bathroom more than usual. It is the same acetoacetate that helps in assuring the level of ketosis with a urine sample test.

Higher Energy Level: If you can cross the initial low phase of the Keto diet, the rest of the experience makes you feel highly energetic. The initial low feeling is also called the Keto flu, which stays for the initial period of the diet. As the body starts utilizing fat for fuel, you get your energy level back. In fact, the produced ketones further enhance the activeness of your brain cells. Hence, you can think better and make decisions faster.

Reduction in Hunger: The fat stored in your body begins to provide regular energy for the body. Once the cycle is created, your body declines the need for food. Hence, many Keto diet followers inform about the reduction in hunger level. This also generates the condition of fasting and further increases the weight loss activity.

Heart Palpitations: You may begin to feel 'fluttery' as a result of dehydration or because of an insufficient intake of salt. Try to adjust, but if you don't feel better quickly, you should seek emergency care.

Disrupted Sleep: The restless night is also a typical side effect. Vitamin supplements can sometimes remedy the problem that can be caused by a lowered insulin and serotonin level. For a quick fix; try 1/2 of a tablespoon of fruit spread and a square of chocolate.

Induction Flu: The diet can make you irritable, nauseous, a bit confused or lethargic, and possibly suffer from a headache. Several days into the plan should remedy these effects. If not, add 1/2 teaspoon of salt to a glass of water, and drink it to help with the side effects. You may need to do this once a day for about the first week, and it could take about 15 to 20 minutes before it helps. It will go away!

Leg Cramps: The loss of magnesium (a mineral) can be a demon and create a bit of pain with the onset of the Keto diet plan changes. With the loss of the minerals during urination, you could experience bouts of cramps in your legs.

Constipation: During the Ketogenic plan, you must drink plenty of water. You can quickly become constipated because of dehydration. The low carbs contribute to the issue. Eat the right veggies and add a small amount of salt to your food to help with the movements. If all else fails, try some Milk of Magnesia.

Checking Ketone Levels

In order to achieve ketosis, you need to have serum ketones between 0.5 and 3.0mM. Below are easy to use home kits to know your ketone levels.

Blood Ketone Meter: It serves as the best and most accurate technique of measuring Beta-Hydroxybutyrate. Blood ketone meters can determine, with precision, the level of ketones in the blood; however, they are quite expensive. The meter costs around $40 and each test strip costs $5. This means that if you want to measure your ketone levels daily, you will need to part with $50.

Breathalyzer: As mentioned earlier, when on a Ketogenic diet, your breath has a distinct smell. A Breathalyzer is a cheap way to measure the concentration of acetone. Keep in mind though that breath ketones can vary from blood ketones.

Urine Test / Urine Ketone Strips: This is one way to measure your ketones for the purpose of ascertaining whether you are in ketosis. Using urine strips, you can easily and simply determine your ketosis without much cost. Testing your urine will readily reveal to you if you have gone over the roof top by eating higher than recommended carbs. Once you dip the stick into your urine, it will turn purple indicating the presence of ketones in your body. A good result for the presence of ketones is dark purple color. When no precise color is shown, it means that you might not have entered ketosis yet.

Ketosis and other urine detection strips may not be as effective because they only show the excess ketone bodies being excreted from the body through the urine. However, they are easy to use and affordable.

Observation: It is possible to know you have attained ketosis by taking a moment listening to the body. For instance, when in ketosis, your breath, urine and sweat smell of acetone, which is a "fruity" smell. If you detect this, then you are most likely in ketosis.

With that understanding of what happens to your body during ketosis, the question you may want to ask is; how then do you get started on the diet?

Chapter 3:
Keto Nutritional Break Down

Being in ketosis is all dependent on consuming the right types of nutrients, the right amounts, and eating those nutrients from the right sources. Let's start with the right types of nutrients. The foods we eat are categorized into different "macronutrients" (more casually known as "macros" if you want to freshen-up your food lingo!). The three main macros are carbs, protein, and fat. If you want to reach Ketosis, then you really need to pay close attention to your macros. Too many carbs and you'll blow your chances, too many proteins and you can really slow the process or stop it all together.

For those of you who've been on the Keto Diet for even a few months, it is clear why these three nutrients are important. They each provide nutrition and energy to your cells that you can't get without consuming them.

1. Carbs
Carbohydrates are most commonly recognized as "starchy" foods such as bread, pasta, potatoes, and rice. However, carbohydrates include sugars and sugar-containing foods such as fruit, candy, cakes,

alcohol... you name it. When you ingest carbs, the body turns them into glucose (blood sugar), which is then used for energy. As soon as the amount of sugar in the blood is raised, your pancreas gets the message to pump out more insulin, so the blood sugar can be processed and moved around the body as energy.

2. Protein

Together with the good fats, protein is one of your body's primary sources of fuel! You can either eat animal proteins, such as meat, fish, eggs, and seafood, or plant protein that's found in nuts, beans, and quinoa. Your brain requires massive amounts of protein for all its processing and daily functions. Protein is very similar to a general handyman, repairing and rebuilding your tissues, making enzymes for better digestion, making hormones (which is what it also does in your brain), and contributes towards building many new cells in your body for things like your muscles, skin, blood, cartilage, and bones. Together with being a fuel source, you can see why it's very important for your body.

3. Fat

Fat is the most important Macro on the Keto Diet, and the most misunderstood, falsely accused, misaligned, and just plain hated. "Fat" is just a short-term nickname for the fatty acids that are present in fats. Fatty acids are long chains of molecules with different chemical components that are various combinations of three atoms: carbon, hydrogen, and oxygen.

There are two types of fats that are lurking in the foods present at your grocery store or served at restaurants:

- *Good Fats*

- *Bad Fats*

Basically, the good fats give you amazing energy, improve your good cholesterol, benefit insulin levels, and control your blood sugar. The bad fats do the opposite. They contribute towards weight gain, raise your bad LDL cholesterol levels, create inflammation, block your arteries, and contribute towards other chronic conditions.

How do you know which fat is your friend and which is your enemy? Read on below to tell the difference.

Good Fats

Saturated Fats – The fatty acid molecules are saturated with hydrogen atoms, thus giving these good fats their name. You can find saturated fats in animal products like meats and dairy. On the Keto Diet, you want to be consuming naturally occurring saturated fats from animals only.

Monounsaturated Fats – These fatty acids only have one double bond that links carbon atoms to hydrogen atoms. These fats don't have as many calories as the saturated fats, so you'd want to eat more of them. They do protect against cardiovascular disease though. Saturated fats come from animal sources, while monoun-saturated fats come from plant sources – nuts, avocados, olive oil, etc.

Natural Polyunsaturated Fats – The processed version of these fatty acids is very bad for you, but the naturally occurring version is great! They're called different names like Omega-3 and Omega-6 fatty acids. You can get your Omega-3 and Omega-6 from walnuts, spinach, eggs, chia seeds, salmon, broccoli, and pumpkin seeds. All those foods are Keto Diet friendly, so eat up!

Bad Fats

Processed Saturated Fats – In addition to naturally occurring saturated fats, these fats can also be created in a laboratory and put into processed foods. That's why they go on the naughty list. Only get your saturated fats from animal sources like meat, dairy, eggs, and seafood.

Processed Polyunsaturated Fats – The natural version is good, but the processed polyunsaturated fats aren't good. If you avoid corn oil, soybean oil, margarine, and those types of foods, you won't be consuming these bad fats. That's why it is important to only buy Ketogenic Diet friendly ingredients and leave these bad fat sources on the shelf.

Trans Fats – Trans-fatty acids are the worst kinds of fats! These are the bad apples that spoil the bunch, because there are so many sources of good fats. But you've got to stay away from these ones.

They were created by the food industry and aren't found naturally occurring in sources from animals or plants. They're like a Frankenstein laboratory experiment gone wrong! If you eat even a small amount of trans fats, your bad cholesterol levels will rise, and you'll be more prone to disease. Trans fats are mostly found in fried or processed foods. Beware!

Fats which are "whole" or "from the source" such as eggs, grass-fed meats, heavy cream, butter, fresh fatty fish such as salmon are all healthy sources of fat. Products which have been processed and refined down to a "different" form than how they started are "bad" fats such as: margarine and vegetable oils (apart from olive oil).

A typical Keto diet, also known as a "long-chain triglyceride diet" usually ensures a consumption ratio of about 3 to 4 grams of fat for every 1 gram of carbohydrate and protein.

In order to ensure you are taking in the accurate levels of each macro, you should track your daily nutrient levels. The general rule is that your daily food should fit within these macro guidelines:

- Fats: 75% of your daily calories

- Protein: 20% of your daily calories

- Carbs: 5% of your daily calories

You may be wondering, what is the timeframe for one to enter ketosis? After 2 days of consuming 20 grams of carbs or less, most people will enter ketosis. Time taken may be, depending on body type, diet plan, and timing of eating.

If you are curious to know about how you can maximize your efforts to fully boost up your Ketosis levels, then all you need to do is follow these simple guidelines.

- Keep your daily carbohydrate intake below 20 carbs.

- Keep your protein levels at around 70g per day.

- Don't starve! Swallow adequate level of fat. Remember that the body is going to need fat to burn fat.

- Try to avoid snack times and stick to your breakfast, lunch and dinner meals with nothing in between.

Chapter 4:
Keto Meats and Nuts Products

You know that you can enjoy beef, bacon, chicken, lamb, cheese, and butter on the Ketogenic diet. So, in this portion, we are going to look at some of the animal-based products that need more recognition for their health benefits.

Sardines are tasty and accessible. If you want a quick meal, you simply must take a can off the shelf and warm it up in the oven for five minutes. Despite this, many people often reach for other canned fish, such as tuna instead. But, while tuna may have its benefits, you are greatly missing out on sardines. One of the great things about sardines is that because they are so small, they eat plankton and no other smaller fish. This leads to them having much less heavy metal toxicity and mercury than fish such as tuna. These fish are a great source of antioxidants, selenium, magnesium, calcium, iron, phosphorous, niacin, vitamin B12, vitamin D, and omega-3s. This leads to sardines being able to help lower cholesterol, increase metabolism, treat gum disease, lower inflammation, improve mental health, strengthen bones, increase energy, and more.

Liver from chicken, beef, duck, and other animals used to be quite popular in order not to waste food. But with the use of supermarkets and the ability to buy select cuts of meat, liver has largely fallen out of favor in America. This is disappointing since it contains many nutrients and health benefits. In fact, the number of nutrients in this small product is amazing. Some of the most potent nutrients within the liver are iron, vitamin B12, vitamin A, riboflavin, copper, choline, and folate.

This simple piece of meat can boost the immune system, increase eye health, increase cellular health and functioning, prevent anemia, increase heart and kidney health, promote the growth of new healthier cells, increase brain function, improve the absorption of iron, boost liver health, and increase energy.

Salmon may not be underappreciated, but many Americans still do not eat enough of this vital fish. Salmon is one of the healthiest fishes and one of the healthiest foods of any type to eat. One of the reasons for this is the large amount of omega-3 fatty acids within salmon. When purchasing salmon, it is best to get wild-caught when possible. This is because farm-raised salmon contains less omega-3s than wild-caught. Studies have found that by eating as little as two servings of salmon a week, we can reach the minimum amount of omega-3 needs.

Salmon is also high in many important B vitamins, selenium, potassium, and antioxidants. It has been found to help lower inflammation, reduce weight, protect against heart disease, protect brain health, and more.

Nuts are a wonderful part of the Ketogenic diet for people without allergies. But it is important to understand how they fit in. Otherwise, it could be easy to cause a stall in your weight loss. While nuts are high in nutrients and much higher in fats than carbs, it's important to realize that their carb count does add up. In fact, cashews, chestnuts, and pistachios are all too high in net carbs to be eaten on the Ketogenic diet. This is especially true because nuts add up quickly. While only an ounce is the serving, people often eat much more than this at any one time. But if you keep an eye on your serving size and how frequently you are eating nuts, you should be fine. However, if you do experience a stall in weight loss for multiple weeks in a row, you might want to cut back on nuts and dairy.

There are many reasons to enjoy pecans. One of the reasons is because they are the lowest nut in net carbs with an ounce containing only 1.1 net carbs. But there are other reasons as well. Pecans are not only the highest nut in antioxidants, but the USDA has even ranked it within the top fifteen antioxidant-rich foods. You can also receive many vitamins and minerals from these nuts, such as selenium, iron, manganese, calcium, zinc, magnesium, and potassium.

Pecans are high in oleic acid, the same type of fat within olives and avocados that give them their signature heart health promoting effect. They can improve digestion, lower cholesterol, reduce the risk of breast and colon cancer, boost the immune system, lower inflammation, treat skin conditions, and slow down aging.

Brazil nuts are a great source of vitamin E, certain B vitamins, magnesium, calcium, and zinc. But what they are best known for is their amazingly high concentration of selenium. In fact, these nuts are the highest known source of this vital nutrient. This micronutrient is an antioxidant and mineral that we require for hormone and immune health, and it helps to protect both our nervous system and cells. Selenium deficiency is well known to be a cause of hyperthyroidism and even sometimes mood disorders such as depression and anxiety. But, by supplementing your diet with natural sources of selenium, you may be able to manage the symptoms or completely recover from these conditions. Eating as few as five or six Brazil nuts can provide you with a full day's serving of selenium.

Macadamia nuts, while may be called a nut, are a seed. But, nonetheless, this nut contains a surprising number of health-promoting monounsaturated fats, magnesium, potassium, selenium, manganese, zinc, calcium, iron, B vitamins, and fiber. One of the types of fat in macadamia nuts is palmitoleic acid. This type of fat is an omega 7, which is incredibly rare but has many benefits. For instance, around our neurons, we have a protective fatty coating, known as myelin.

When this myelin begins to become damaged, it leads to symptoms of neurodegenerative diseases and mental illness. But, palmitoleic acid is a major component of our myelin, meaning that by eating more through macadamia nuts can promote our neurological health. As if that weren't enough to boost our brain, their contents of thiamine, copper, and iron are all essential for brain health.

Walnuts have long been centered in medical research for their many amazing properties. In fact, every year there is a medical conference at the University of California detailing all the latest research on this powerful nut. There is a good reason to choose walnuts; they are higher in antioxidant activity and omega-3 fats than any of the other nuts. The antioxidants from the plant compounds, vitamin E, and melatonin have many benefits, including lowering bad cholesterol and improving heart health. With the high number of omega-3s in walnuts, you can gain two and a half grams for each one-ounce serving.

The plant compounds within walnuts, known as polyphenols, have many benefits. One of these benefits is that they directly target inflammation and oxidative damage that is the direct cause of many illnesses. This means that they can directly impact cancer, Alzheimer's disease, diabetes, autoimmune diseases, neurological diseases, and more. Studies have also found that by consuming walnuts regularly, we may be able to lower high blood pressure.

Hazelnuts, also known as filberts, like many nuts are high in healthy fats and antioxidants. This nut has specifically been the focus of many studies on inflammation and how it leads to disease. In study after study, it has found that the antioxidants within hazelnuts, known as phenolic compounds, can greatly reduce inflammation. This, in turn, can help protect against cancer, neurodegenerative diseases, and more. Although, it's important to know that most of the antioxidants found within hazelnuts are within the skin of the nut. Not only that, but by roasting the nut prior to eating it, the number of antioxidants is reduced. Therefore, it is best to enjoy these nuts raw and with the skin intact.

Almonds may be higher in nuts than the others we have discussed so far, but they are still low enough to be eaten in moderation on the Ketogenic diet. In fact, products such as almond milk make a wonderful addition when you are on a Keto lifestyle. These nuts are high in vitamin E, manganese, phosphorus, calcium, iron, magnesium, antioxidants, and fiber. They have been shown to manage blood pressure, lower cholesterol, improve heart health, increase brain health, and promote strong bones and teeth.

Chia seeds are a small black seed that only recently took the world by storm due to their powerful nutrients. But despite only recently coming into the focus of health-conscious people, these seeds have a long and rich history with the Mayans and Aztecs. Part of the reason these seeds are so amazing is that despite their tiny size, they hold an incredible amount of nutrients. In fact, a single ounce of chia seeds contains only one-hundred and thirty-seven calories and two net carbs. This means that calorie for calorie, chia seeds are one of the best nutrient sources in the world. A few of the nutrients these seeds contain are phosphorous, manganese, zinc, B vitamins, magnesium, potassium, and omega-3 fatty acids. Of course, they also hold quite a few antioxidants, as well. In a single ounce of chia, you can also gain four grams of protein and eight grams of healthy fats.

These seeds can help with weight loss, improve heart health, strengthen bones, lower inflammation levels, balance blood sugar, and more.

While sesame seeds may be tiny and overlooked, they are a rich source of healthy fats, antioxidants, fiber, magnesium, iron, calcium, potassium, phosphorous, zinc, copper, vitamin E, and certain B vitamins. These seeds have been shown to improve heart health, reduce the risk of certain cancers, prevent diabetes, increase bone strength, reduce male infertility, manage blood pressure, increase heart health, reduce inflammation, treat respiratory diseases, improve dental health, increase blood circulation, and much more. A single ounce of sesame seeds contains one-hundred and sixty calories, thirteen grams of healthy fats, five grams of protein, and three net carbs.

Flaxseeds are commonly used in low-carb baking. After all, a single ounce only contains half of a net carb while also having five grams of protein and eleven grams of heart-healthy fat. But these seeds have more benefits than their low-carb proprieties. Flaxseeds are full of omega-3 fatty acids, fiber, potassium, magnesium, calcium, iron, phosphorous, and certain B vitamins as well.

Flaxseeds are full of lignans, a plant compound and antioxidant which has been shown to greatly reduce the risk of both breast cancer and prostate cancer. In fact, flaxseeds contain up to eight-hundred times more lignans than other plants. One study of over six-thousand women found that those who regularly eat flaxseeds are eighteen percent less likely to develop breast cancer. Along with their anti-cancer benefits, these seeds also lower cholesterol, lower high cholesterol, and manage blood sugar.

Chapter 5:
Keto Vegetable Products

There is a reason that parents have long told children to eat their broccoli. Whether this cruciferous vegetable is eaten steamed or raw, it has many health benefits. In fact, some people even label broccoli as a 'superfood' due to it being an amazing source of vitamins - A, E, C, K, B vitamins, iron, calcium, selenium potassium, and fiber.

One of these vitamins, vitamin K, is essential for the natural clotting process in our blood as well as bone health and strength. Studies have even shown that if we increase our consumption of vitamin K, we may prevent osteoporosis and fractures as we age. We can easily consume more than our recommended intake with a single serving of broccoli. This makes broccoli a wonderful addition to your daily diet.

Broccoli: As if those weren't all good reasons to include broccoli on the Ketogenic diet, a single cup of this vegetable is only four net carbs. Whether you eat broccoli with Ranch dressing, cheese sauce, butter, bacon, or on its own, you are sure to find a way you can fully enjoy this vegetable ripe with benefits.

Kale and Spinach: Eating dark leafy greens is important, we all know that. Therefore, kale and spinach are so very popular. Kale and spinach taste different, but what about the nutritional differences? Firstly, both vegetables are full of vitamins and minerals. They have been shown to improve our cardiovascular health, immune system, bone health, and prevention of diseases as we age. The high content of vitamin C within these vegetables can even help our skin to age better.

Out of both vegetables, kale is higher in calories and carbohydrates. One hundred grams of kale contains forty-nine calories and five net carbohydrates whereas the same amount of spinach contains twenty-three calories and one net carb. That is quite a difference in carbohydrates. But kale is also higher in calcium and both vitamins K and A.

Mushroom; Mushrooms are commonly known as a superfood. This is because half of all edible mushrooms can benefit our health more than on just a basic nutritional need. They are known as a functional food because they can directly prevent and treat illnesses and disease. This has been shown to be true in both scientific studies and in practice for thousands of years in ancient Chinese medicine. This fungus contains antiviral, antibacterial, and ironically antifungal properties. They have also been shown to treat and reduce the risk of cancer, manage blood pressure, lower inflammation, strengthen the immune system, improve hair and skin health, lower cholesterol, and more.

Mushrooms are a tasty addition to the Ketogenic diet and incredibly low in carbohydrates. One-hundred ounces of white button mushrooms only contains two net carbohydrates.

Asparagus: Asparagus may be a popular vegetable, but did you know that it is part of the lily family? These little spears have many benefits, which are especially wonderful since one-hundred grams only contains about two net carbs. Asparagus is high in vitamins K, A, C, E, and B9 as well as phosphorous, fiber, potassium, and antioxidants. Studies have shown that this vegetable can improve your digestive health, nutrient absorption, cholesterol levels, manage blood pressure, and support a healthy pregnancy. Whether you are enjoying green, white, or purple asparagus, you will receive many benefits.

Bell Peppers: Bell peppers may be higher in carbs per gram than some options, but when enjoyed in moderation they are low enough to be fully enjoyed on the Ketogenic diet. This is great because they are also high in many nutrients. You can find one of the richest sources of vitamin C in bell peppers, along with vitamins K, B6, B9, E, and vitamin A as well as potassium. One bell pepper, or forty-five grams, contains four net carbs. This nightshade can help to reduce the risk of heart disease and cancer, boost the immune system, increase eye health, slow down aging, increase cognitive health, and promote a healthy pregnancy.

Green Beans: While beans are not usually allowed on the Ketogenic diet, green beans are the exception. These are young pole or bush beans that are extremely high in fiber and low in carbohydrates. In fact, while one-hundred grams of pinto beans contains forty-seven net carbohydrates, the same amount of green beans only contains four. They serve as wonderful sources for vitamin C, A, B6, K, fiber, calcium, iron, manganese, copper, potassium, and folic acid as well. The antioxidants within these beans have been shown to improve heart health and reduce the risk of developing heart disease. They also reduce the risk of colon cancer, boost the immune system, manage diabetes, strengthen bone health, improve eye health, treat gastrointestinal disorders, and improve pregnancy health.

Zucchini: The possibilities of cooking with zucchini are nearly limitless. One of many people's favorite ways to use this summer squash on the Ketogenic diet is to put it through a spiralizer and turn it into "noodles." These noodles can be made into a long list of pasta dishes at a fraction of the calorie and carb count. Actually, one-hundred grams of zucchini only contains two net carbs. This vegetable can also manage blood sugar, improve digestion, increase eye health, slow down aging, increase heart health, improve adrenal and thyroid functioning, lower inflammation, and boost energy levels.

Spaghetti Squash: Like zucchini, spaghetti squash can easily be made into low-carb pasta dishes. In fact, many people will roast and then stuff spaghetti squash with their favorite pasta toppings creating a decadent meal. One-hundred grams of this winter squash contains six net carbs. They are high in fiber and vitamins A, C, K, B9, as well as manganese. They are known to boost the immune system, reduce inflammation, increase lung health, manage blood circulation, strengthen bones, and much more.

Chapter 6:
Keto Fruits, Dairy, and Oil Products

Most fruits are high in glucose and fructose, causing a blood sugar spike and insulin response. Most are simply too high to be included on the Ketogenic diet. But that doesn't mean you have to forsake all fruits. Berries are an incredibly healthy source of fiber, vitamins, minerals, and antioxidants, all while being low enough in carbs to enjoy on the Ketogenic diet.

Strawberry: Strawberries are known to be a great source of vitamin C, vitamin B9 (folate), potassium, manganese, and antioxidants. This has been shown to improve the immune system, regulate blood sugar, lowers the risk of vision defects/cataracts, protect against cancer, treat arthritis, manage mood, lower allergic reaction severity, and more. One-hundred grams of strawberries contains six net carbohydrates.

Blueberry: Blueberries are higher in carbohydrates than strawberries, and therefore you are more limited in how many you can enjoy. Yet, they have many health benefits and are another good addition to the Ketogenic diet. This little berry is particularly high in fiber, manganese, vitamin C, vitamin K, and antioxidants. They are known to reduce cellular damage to our DNA, manage blood pressure, improve brain health and memory, reduce muscle damage, prevent heart disease, and more. These berries contain twice the number of net carbs as strawberries, with fifty grams containing six net carbs.

Olive: There are many benefits to eating olives, whether in their natural form or in the form of extra virgin olive oil. Many people may think that they are a vegetable, but they are in fact a fruit. While some have vaguely heard that olive oil is healthy, most haven't taken the time to learn its many health benefits. Worse yet, most people on the standard American diet eat a large portion of trans fats and fats with no nutritional properties rather than the amazing fats found in olives. Yet, this fruit has been shown to be high in antioxidants that protect against cancer, improve digestion, increase blood circulation, reduce inflammation, lower allergic reactions, increase brain function, reverse bone loss, manage blood pressure, and protect against infections.

This fruit is also high in essential omega-3 fatty acids, iron copper, sodium, calcium, and vitamin E. If you are interested in adding whole olives to your diet in addition to olive oil, you will be happy to know that a one-hundred-gram serving only contains three net carbs with ten grams of health-promoting fats.

Avocado: Avocados are one of the Ketogenic power foods. Sure, you can fully enjoy the Keto diet without avocados. But, the healthy fat, nutrient-dense, and low-carb fruit is the ideal of the Keto pyramid. One-hundred grams of this fruit, about half of a Haas avocado, only contains two net carbs. When eating avocados, you will be getting plenty of potassium, fiber, antioxidants, healthy fats, and vitamins K, B9, B5, B6, and E. In fact, while some people may be worried that bananas are non-Ketogenic and what that will mean for their potassium levels, avocados are much higher in potassium than a banana.

Dairy Products: Make use of dairy products such as yogurt, sour cream, cottage cheese, goat cheese, and whole milk.

I am a big fan of lard and olive oil (extra virgin) as they cook well and make food taste fantastic. Lard is good for the body. There are 12 grams of fat per serving, but only 5 grams of saturated fat. About half the fat in lard is Monounsaturated - you know the kind of fat that supposedly makes olive oil good for us. The saturated fat, of course, will primarily raise your HDL levels and that is a good thing if you ask me. The fatty-acid profile of lard is very similar to human body fat. And if you lose weight and consume your own fat in the process, that's good for you.

Butter is great, added salt or unsalted is fine. Stay away from fake butters such as margarine and vegetable oil butters, except if it is olive oil butter, however it must be 100% olive oil not 40 percent and the rest vegetable oil. I tell you to stay away from make believe butter not because they contain carbs but because of that pesky trans-fat (hydrogenated oils) that have been getting talked about lately. They are seriously not good for you and should not be included in anyone's diet. Extra-virgin olive oil is unrefined, low in fats and contains lots of antioxidants.

When it comes to the fat on the meat please do not remove the valuable fat off like a surgeon, not only will the food taste bland but you're missing out on precious fats' ability to help you burn up stored body fat. So, keep the steak fat on, the chicken skin, and bacon strips fat also. Remember we're not following the low-fat dogma high carbohydrate diet anymore.

Coconut oil boosts metabolism and ketosis. Grass-fed butter and ghee have lots of nutrients, antibiotics and good for use when on Keto diet. You may also use sesame oil and avocado oil.

Chapter 7:
Well Formulated Ketogenic Meals

Breakfasts

- Pancakes, made with eggs and cream cheese (add a little almond flour if you don't like the texture)

- Eggs

- Bacon

- Sausage

- Check the ingredients and avoid any added fillers such as rusk.

- Be careful of the ingredients in vegetarian sausages. Avoid those that have a high grain and sugar content. Don't worry about the salt at this stage – you need it!

- Mushrooms

- Tomatoes

- Cloud Bread (see the recipe in chapter 7)

Lunch

- Use cream cheese pancakes to roll sandwich ingredients inside, such as ham, cheese, egg, and mayo

- Salads with ingredients such as, lettuce, cucumber, bell peppers, radish, tomatoes

- You can add ingredients such as, tuna, cheese, or eggs to your salads

- Sprinkle seeds on your salad to add a crunchy texture

Dinner Meats

- Chicken drumsticks

- Chicken breast with soy sauce and sesame seeds

- Fish, such as salmon or cod

- Pork chops

- Ground beef

- Beef steaks

Dinner Vegetables

- Cauliflower

- Green leafy vegetables like bok choy, spinach, or chard

Dinner Sauces

- Add extra shredded cheese to cream cheese, then melt together to make a rich sauce

- Use Worcestershire, soy sauce, or mustard to add flavor to your sauces and gravies

Snacks

- Beef or chicken broth

- Avocado

- Around 10 nuts

- Unprocessed string cheese

Drinks

- Coffee with full-fat cream

- Green tea

- Water with lemon slices

- If you sweeten your drinks, use an alternative natural sweetener such as Stevia or Erythritol

- Red wine in the recommended moderation - you will need to deduct this from your carb count for the day

Chapter 8:
Finding Your Carb Sweet Spot

Most people consider a macronutrient breakdown of fat at 62%, protein at 28% while carbs stand at 10%. You can always cut down on carbs and protein to ensure that you burn more fat.

There are reasons why you need to trim down on protein. If you eat excess protein, the body converts it to glucose. In return, the level of blood insulin will rise, making the body to not get rid and burn the fat.

When it comes to the amount of carbs, do not cut the carb levels immediately with the intention of attaining your weight loss sweet spot. You can change to something closer to 30 to 50g net carbs each day and have a spike of 100 – 130g net carbs once or two times in each week. This can be an awesome formula to ensure that you are in line with your weight loss goals. But if you aim at losing 20 to 25 pounds, you need to eat less than 20g of net carbs in a day.

You can aim at daily ration of 75% fat, 20% protein and 5% carbs. To get your sweet spot, include such items like leaf and fat lard, ghee, unprocessed beef tallow and coconut oil. Enjoy the grass-fed types of meat.

Do not cut on carbs drastically. Reduce the count slowly like around 40 to 50g until you attain your sweet spot.

Chapter 9:
Intermittent Fasting

In today's modern food culture, we have been conditioned for the entirety of our lives that we need to eat throughout the day to keep our bodies healthy. It commonly known that breakfast is a vital meal to kickstart the day, or that eating small meals every 2-3 hours is ideal for an efficient metabolism. The truth is, eating with this kind of frequency is not the way our species were made to function, and is a relatively new trend amongst humans.

By giving the body a break, such as following the intermittent fasting lifestyle, we can become a healthier, more efficient physical machine that performs at the level it was designed for. So, what is Intermittent Fasting? Answering this question is probably a good idea before we discuss any further details about it. Intermittent Fasting, put simply, is a diet protocol in which you do not eat throughout the day, only consuming all your daily calories within a specific eating window that you designate. The time that you spend fasting throughout the day is usually far longer than the eating window.

The key aspect to point out here is that you are not consuming any CALORIES during the fasting period, you are still free to consume as much water as you need (very important), as well as any flavored drinks or dietary supplements that you choose as long as they are calorie free. For example, most people that adhere to intermittent fasting engage in a 16-hour fast day, followed by an 8-hour eating window. One of the benefits of this protocol is that you can decide on your eating window based on your lifestyle, making intermittent fasting very convenient.

If you are an early bird, being most productive early in the day and usually in bed when the sun goes down, you can choose to eat earlier, say from 9am-5pm. For all the night owls out there, who see midnight on a regular basis, pushing you're eating window back to 4pm-12am is not a problem at all. Any way you design your intermittent fasting plan is fine, so long as you follow the foundational rules: no calories during your fasting period (while still staying properly hydrated) and sticking to consuming all your calories during the strict eating window that you designate.

If you are hearing intermittent fasting for the first time, you may be ready to close it immediately and never even consider this lifestyle. If that is you, this feeling is probably due to outdated fitness and nutrition advice that society and so-called "gurus" have hammered into your mind for decades. You have without a doubt heard that breakfast is the most important meal of the day, or eating 5-6 small meals every 2-3 hours throughout the day is the most effective way for efficient metabolism, or that 'starving' yourself to lose weight is counterproductive, etc.

Before we even begin to debunk these myths with all the benefits of intermittent fasting, you need to realize that this is not a new concept by any means. Eating throughout the course of the entire day is a relatively new concept. Food has become so convenient and accessible today that we are trained into believing we need three square meals a day. Society is so concerned with eating, instant gratification of our dietary desires that there are fast food restaurants on every corner with their flashing neon signs advertising the latest $5 calorie bomb. Is it any surprise then, that obesity levels are soaring, heart disease and stroke are running rampant, and people are unhealthier than ever before?

From our earliest ancestors all the way up until a few hundred years ago, the habit of eating one large meal at the end the day was the norm. Ancient humans were hunter-gatherers, spending the entire day foraging for edible vegetation, hunting game, and just trying to survive. Eating was considered a celebratory ritual and was accompanied by a feast each evening when the food was brought back to the tribe. Even our modern ancestors spent their days farming the land, working whatever job needed to be done for their families, eating one large meal after a hard day's work.

While I am by no means saying that these people had it better than we do now (I would rather eat a few too many calories each day than have to survive a saber-toothed tiger attack), they did in fact reap many of the benefits of intermittent fasting without even realizing it. To digress, eating throughout the duration of the day is a relatively new concept that is not at all necessary to a healthy lifestyle.

So, what exactly is intermittent fasting and why does it work? Intermittent Fasting (IF) may just be the best-kept secret of the diet and fitness industry. With over 100 years of research to back up this amazing game changing lifestyle, intermittent fasting is poised to take the health and wellness community by storm.

Before we jump into what intermittent fasting is, and why it works, let's first go over a couple of things that intermittent fasting is not.

First, intermittent fasting is NOT a diet plan. There are no off-limits foods, no meal plans, no meal prepping, and no complicated recipes. In fact, you can practice intermittent fasting and eat whatever you want. You'll still get some of the benefits. Of course, intermittent fasting works best when you try to eat more vegetables and whole foods, while eating less processed foods. It isn't necessary, and you can keep having treats without any guilt.

Second, intermittent fasting is NOT a metabolism lowering calorie restriction game. In fact, intermittent fasting can be used to lose weight, maintain weight, or even gain muscle. What does this mean for you? If you like intermittent fasting, and it ends up being a good fit, you can practice it for the rest of your life. It helps you lose weight, of course, but it has so many more benefits than just that.

Intermittent Fasting: The Basics

Let's get down to it. What is intermittent fasting? In short, intermittent fasting is a pattern of eating that involves periods of fasting, and periods of feasting. If this sounds frightening, don't worry! You've already been practicing the traditional eating pattern for your whole life.

This is what you've probably been taught: breakfast is the most important meal of the day, and you need to eat it about 30 minutes to 1-hour after you wake up. Your day should consist of three large meals, and two snacks. Many individuals have been made to believe this eating pattern is the best for our health.

But what if there was a body of research out there that proved otherwise? What if I told you that by not eating for periods of 16, 24, or even 36 hours, you could lose weight, gain muscle, and boost your energy levels and overall health? Well this is all true, and it's called intermittent fasting.

There are several different methods of intermittent fasting, and you will learn how to incorporate the top four in a later chapter. For now, let's just go over the basics. To practice intermittent fasting, you don't eat for 16+ hours. For most people, that means eating dinner at

7pm, going to sleep, and then not eating again until lunch the next day. Not eating for 16 hours might sound hard, but it becomes a lot easier if you sleep through 8 of those hours!

You may already have practiced intermittent fasting without realizing it. Have you ever woken up late on the weekend, or met a friend for a late brunch around noon? If that is your first meal of the day, you're practicing intermittent fasting.

If your first reaction to this is reluctance, keep reading. Over the next chapters, we will discuss why intermittent fasting is the right lifestyle for you and how you can easily integrate it into your life.

However, you may think to yourself, I'll be so hungry if I skip breakfast! We'll get more into this later, but after the first week or two, you really won't feel hungry! Your mind is used to eating in the morning, so for the first week, you will feel hungry. Once your brain learns to wait until lunch for food that hunger will go away. In many ways, intermittent fasting teaches you to listen to your body more closely.

The Science Behind the Lifestyle

To convince ourselves that intermittent fasting really is the lifestyle choice for us, let's go over a few of the scientific reasons why intermittent fasting causes weight loss without damaging our metabolism.

It is important to understand how chemistry that is external to our bodies has an impact on our fat loss and storage. Because when we say we want to lose weight, we mean that we want to lose fat. Now, most people follow the "calories in, calories out" method of weight loss. When you ingest fewer calories as compared to what you burn, you will lose weight. While this is true, researchers have now shown us that it leaves our metabolisms low, and we are almost guaranteed to put the weight back on.

Intermittent Fasting works because it doesn't rely on the calories in, calories out equation to promote weight loss. Instead, intermittent fasting prompts fat loss by lowering our insulin levels. So, how does insulin work?

Intermittent Fasting and Your Body's Chemistry

Insulin tells our body when it is time to store energy as fat, and when it is time to burn fat as energy. When we eat, our stomach and liver turn food into energy. Some of that energy goes into our blood stream as blood sugar, and we use that immediately. The rest? Stored as fat.

Insulin is a chemical, released by our pancreas when we eat, that tells our body it is time to store fat. So, when we don't eat for 16 hours or more, our insulin level goes down significantly, and our body transitions into the fat burning mode. So, even if you ate a large dinner the night before, you'll still go into fat burning mode the next morning!

Insulin isn't the only chemical that a fast trigger, however. When we fast for longer than 16 hours, our body produces more human growth hormone (HGH). This fantastic hormone tells our body to burn fat, repair muscle, and even build new muscles! By fasting, you will lose weight and have more energy!

Yet there is even one more reason that intermittent fasting kicks the calories in calories out method of weight loss: when you fast for over 16 hours, your body produces more adrenaline. Adrenaline, in turn, gives you more energy and mental awareness! You'll feel energetic and thoughtful even when you haven't eaten recently.

The combination of these three effects, lower insulin, increased HGH, and increased adrenaline, combine in your body to raise your metabolism, sometimes up to 14% higher than your base rate. This boost in metabolism can lead to some great weight loss results! You will also be reducing your calories somewhat, since you eat fewer meals each day. This slight calorie reduction, plus increased metabolism, will lead to fantastic and long-lasting results.

How IF Works

For you to understand how intermittent fasting works, it is important to understand how the body processes the food you eat.

When you eat (if you follow the USDA's food pyramid, which entails high carb, minimal fat and moderate protein intake), the body goes into a fed state i.e. a state in which the body has high levels of various nutrients in the bloodstream. The fed state lasts for about 3-5 hours after which your body goes into a post-absorptive state where nothing is being digested although the levels of insulin are still high in the blood. This is the time the cells are taking up any remaining blood glucose for use or storage. During this period (the fed state and post absorptive state, the body is actively digesting everything you've eaten so that some can be absorbed into the bloodstream for transportation to different parts of the body where the cells in various parts use them for energy.

After the food is absorbed and is in the bloodstream for transportation to different parts of the body, one challenge arises though; the cells don't have their own mechanism for absorbing glucose from the bloodstream. In fact, they can only do that with the aid of insulin, a hormone secreted by the pancreas in response to rising blood glucose concentrations. The purpose of insulin is simple; to 'open the gates' to the cells so that they can take up the glucose in the bloodstream in order to maintain a healthy level of blood glucose concentration. This essentially means that even if there is an excess of blood glucose (after the fed state), the presence of insulin in the bloodstream keeps the 'doors' open so that the cells take up more glucose. They don't use everything though; the excess glucose is first converted into glycogen, which is then stored in the liver.

Glycogen is like an emergency/backup source of energy, which kicks in when glucose levels in the blood are low for an extended period. But the glycogen stores are limited; they can only take about 2000kcal of energy at any given time. So, if there is still an excess of glucose available for the cells, it is converted into fatty acids and glycerol, which are then stored in the various fat stores around the body e.g. around organs, under the skin etc. The thing is; the presence of insulin in the bloodstream tends to promote fat storage and inhibits fat burning.

The entire process i.e. being in the fed state (up to the time the body no longer has any glucose which needs to be used up in the blood-stream) takes about 10-12 hours after you've had your meal. If you don't take any more food, this is when you start entering the fasted state, a state where the body has no more glucose in the bloodstream but is 'hungry' for nutrients. What does it do? Well, it goes to its backup power source i.e. glycogen, which it converts into glucose for use in different body processes with the help of glucagon (another hormone secreted by the pancreas) in the liver. At this time, the body doesn't just break down glycogen exclusively; it starts loosening up its grip on other energy stores e.g. the fat stores so that they can be burned to fuel different body processes. This means when you are in a fasted state (i.e. after 12-14 hours from your last meal), you can be sure of losing weight without struggle. The goal of intermittent fasting is to induce the fasted state by spacing meals in a manner that you get to a fasted state every single day so as to push your body to the point of starting to burn glycogen (and perhaps deplete it a little) so that it can start burning more stored fat for energy.

The challenge with most of us is that we hardly get to the fasted state; we are very used to eating breakfast, lunch and dinner in some predetermined structure. The challenge though is that this 'structure' hardly gets us into a fasted state. In fact, we are always in the fed state, as many of us eat many meals about 4-5 hours apart. Obviously, this results in a nutrient overload and always keeps us in the fed state because this essentially keeps the body in the fed state. It is only after dinner when we try to get to the fasted state while we are asleep. But given that many of us take breakfast quite early and delay our dinner time, we hardly really 'get there.'

Do you know that this has great adverse effects on your body? Well, let me explain.

As you already know, most of the time, our bodies are in the fed state and not the fasted state making our cells more adapted to burning glucose instead of fat for energy. This simply means that normally, the levels of insulin are always high. There is a problem though; with insulin levels always high, the cells start becoming more 'blind' to the signals of insulin such that more insulin is required to trigger the cells to open to take up glucose. This is referred to as insulin resistance. In such a state, the body is always burning glucose and rarely ever burns fat (the presence of insulin has fat burning inhibitory properties) and when the glucose is depleted, the body doesn't move to the fasted stage; instead, it gets hungry for more glucose. This is because the body has less capacity to mobilize and burn fat for energy. So, you can picture the cravings and the excess fat storage that comes with insulin resistance.

The secret to weight loss is in structuring your meals in a manner that ensures you get your 12-14 hours minimum from the time you had your last meal to the next. The rest of the hours i.e. 12-10 hours are up to you; eat whatever you want but just don't overindulge! With fasting, this process goes on reverse. When you don't eat for an extended period, the levels of insulin fall as a result of falling blood glucose levels, which signals the body to burn stored energy (glycogen and fats) since no more is coming in. This brings about weight loss in the long term.

From the above explanation, the period within which you stay without food ought to start from about 12-14 hours (no less). If you want to fast for longer, you are free to do that; this brings about fasted effects because you get to use more of the stored fats for energy. The feeding window therefore is within 10-8 hours or less (not more).

Note: You can increase the fasting hours to achieve greater benefits. To simplify things, you can follow different intermittent fasting protocols, which we will discuss later.

So how exactly does intermittent fasting result to weight loss? Well, there are different explanations to this.

• You effectively create a calorie deficit when you fast.

- You ultimately are likely to consume fewer calories within the feeding window, something which will create the much-needed calorie deficit for weight loss

- You enhance your metabolism with intermittent fasting.

Chapter 10:
Why Try Intermittent Fasting

By following this protocol, you are far more likely to consume fewer calories during the day. The foundation of any weight loss plan is often lost behind complicated diet plans and flawed philosophies that serve to confuse people more than they help them. This foundation is that calories are the key to weight gain or loss. If you consume fewer calories per day than your body burns, you are going to lose weight. Likewise, if you take in a surplus of calories compared to what your body burns, weight gain is inevitable.

What happens when we eat regular meals all throughout the day? You wake up, eat breakfast, and then usually even before lunch you get hungry again, indulging in a snack here and there. After lunch, we usually have a 4-6-hour wait before dinner and then more snacks to satisfy our urges tend to follow. With this constant cycle of eating, getting full, and then getting hungry again and eating more between meals, it makes it so easy for us to consume too many calories throughout the day. With intermittent fasting, once your body adjusts to the prolonged fasting period, you will eat fewer meals because you are limited to a timed 'feeding' window. This allows you to prevent excess hunger between meals and feel relatively satiated throughout the duration.

For example, the average person is advised to follow a 2,000-calorie per day diet. Which one is challenging to achieve, eating throughout the entire day, 3 meals and snacks included, while only consuming 2,000 calories, or only allowing yourself 8 hours to eat the same number? Obviously, it is easier to eat a healthy number of calories if you limit them to a shorter window. Intermittent fasting will allow you to more easily consume your desired number of calories than eating all day will.

Another profound benefit of intermittent fasting is an increase in insulin sensitivity in the body. As we discussed earlier, our society is experiencing an obesity epidemic of epic proportions. Hand in hand with obesity is type 2 diabetes. Type 2 diabetes results when the body is unable to use insulin properly. When this happens, the pancreas (the organ that produces insulin) will attempt to produce extra insulin at first, but will eventually be unable to keep up, causing blood glucose levels to soar.

Obesity is associated with type 2 diabetes due to the fact that when the pancreas has to constantly release a large amount of insulin (typical of a poor diet, a primary cause of obesity), eventually the insulin receptors in the body become overloaded and lose their ability to use insulin efficiently. Almost 90% of the people living with type 2 diabetes are obese or overweight.

As we discuss obesity, losing weight, and burning fat, let's use basic human biology to explain why we store fat in the first place. The human body is an incredible machine, it is designed to survive many hardships, and famine is one of them. When we consume an excess of calories, the body will use as many calories as it needs at the time, but then stores away the rest as either glycogen in the liver, but more readily, as adipose tissue (or fat).

This was extremely necessary for the ancient man, when food was scarce and unavailable for sometimes days on end; the body used the fat it had stored during times of plentiful food to survive. Fat, however, is not the body's go to source for fuel in normal situations. If food is readily available, it will use glucose as a primary energy source, saving the fat for more drastic times. In today's world, with eating all throughout the day is the norm and food more readily available than ever before, the average person's body today tends to get its energy almost exclusively from glucose. We never experience that famine situation in which our fat stores were designed to withstand.

As advanced as we think we've become in our society, it is ironic that our actual genome has changed very little since ancient humans. Even today, if we engage in intermittent fasting, we signal to the body that we are experiencing a period of scarce food and, once the body gets used to this protocol, we see a shift in its primary energy source. By following the intermittent fasting protocol, we can train the body to start using our fat stores for energy instead of glucose alone. Most overweight people today are caught in a cycle where the blood glucose is always elevated due to being full. When this starts to decrease, instead of their body switching to burning fat as fuel, they simply get hungry and eat again. This not only keeps blood glucose way too high consistently, but also does not allow the body to burn fat like it otherwise would.

Another little known but monumental benefit of intermittent fasting is that it has been shown to decrease the odds of contracting breast cancer in women, and aid in the fight against cancer in general once a woman has developed it. A study of 7,000 women with a history of anorexia showed a 50% reduction in the incidence of breast cancer. Before we go any further yes, anorexia is a horrible disease but what researchers took from this was that caloric restriction and fasting, all characteristic of anorexia, decreases breast cancer risks. Intermittent fasting reduces the side effects of chemotherapy and even increase its effectiveness when used immediately before and after chemo.

What an enormous benefit to gain from a change in diet. Literally everything we do with proper nutrition and exercise, goes back to trying to live if we can and be healthy while we are here. Intermittent fasting has consistently shown to increase the lifespan of numerous animals, which is what you and I are as well! Not to mention that living a healthy and happy life is one of the most important things to do while we live on this beautiful planet.

Another positive side effect associated with intermittent fasting is improved brain health. We can agree that the brain is an important organ to look out for, as even agreeing with this statement requires the brain. Prolonged periods of fasting slowed down the flow of information across the neurons in the brain. Although slowing down our brains may seem counter intuitive, this benefits our mental health.

The stress of day-to-day life which we all experience has our neuronal circuits constantly firing, leaving the brain overworked by our tedious schedules. Too much activity in the synapses of the brain, (which are responsible for relaying information) has been linked with several diseases of the brain and nervous system, such as Alzheimer's and Parkinson's disease. It seems as if the slowing down of the brain through fasting gives it a break, allowing it to recharge. When in a fasting state, the body produces compounds known as ketone bodies, which are known to protect the neurons in the brain, preventing them from degrading to the point of disease. Furthermore, intermittent fasting has even been proven extremely effective in combating depression and anxiety.

'Brain-derived neurotrophic factor' is a chemical released in the brain that is responsible for the formation of neuronal networks. In people suffering from depression, we see this chemical suppressed substantially. When these new neuronal networks have a difficult time forming and branching out, depression is far more likely. A study from the Neurobiology of Disease in 2007 concluded that periods of fasting can increase the concentration of Brain-Derived Neurotrophic factor anywhere from 50 to 400 percent! We're not talking about a slight increase here; this is a huge amount.

Another chemical chain that occurs in the brain during periods of fasting and caloric restriction, involves a hormone called Ghrelin. Ghrelin is known as the hunger hormone because it increases when we are hungry and/or fasting. When it comes to mental health, however, increased Ghrelin is very helpful. Not only has this hormone been linked to elevated mood, it is a natural antidepressant and promotes neurogenesis in the brain.

In our world today, chronic depression and anxiety levels are at an all-time high, and people report feeling higher levels of anxiety than ever before. Intermittent fasting is a good consideration to circumvent this trend and help keep your mood uplifted throughout the day. Not only will this lifestyle alter the chemical balance in your brain, allowing you to combat and prevent depression, but the weight-loss and fitness benefits will serve to improve your self-image and confidence, which are both aspects of life that, when negative, cause depression and anxiety. Think of intermittent fasting as a double-edged sword that slices through both obesity and depression.

Intermittent fasting may seem to be a new trend that has emerged in the spotlight recently, as many fad diets plans often do, but rest assured that this is not a recent new way of life. This lifestyle has been around far longer than you and I have been alive, or even our great-great (times 20) grandparents have been around to consider it.

Today's modern food culture has led us to believe that we must not go any more than a few hours without eating, and that our entire day should be based around meals. The science behind intermittent fasting does not agree. Should you choose to give this lifestyle a try, you could reap all the benefits that we've discussed and more. While skipping meals and engaging in a prolonged period of fasting may go against all your prior beliefs on eating and how food should be consumed, I strongly believe that you will find the benefits worth the try.

More About Weight Loss

Your body tends to store energy in the form of fat cells. When you don't eat anything, there a couple of different changes that take place in your body that help your body access its energy reserves, and in the activity of your nervous system. Here are what takes place in the metabolism of your body whenever you fast.

Insulin- The level of insulin increases whenever you eat. So, while you are fasting, the insulin levels in your body will decrease. A low level of insulin means that it is easier for your body to burn the fats that are stored within.

Human Growth Hormone - The human growth hormone or HGH level increases when you fast. This hormone is responsible for not just fat loss, but it also helps with muscle gain and it kick starts autophagy.

Noradrenaline - Norepinephrine or noradrenaline is sent to the fat cells by the nervous system to help break down the fat in the body and to free up the reserves of fatty acids to provide energy.

If you keep consuming food throughout the day, then it is unlikely that any of these changes will take place. Short-term fasting helps increase your body's ability to burn fats. So, a short-term fast like intermittent fasting induces several changes in your body that makes it easier to burn fat. It also reduces the production of insulin while increasing the production of the growth hormone and epinephrine to give a metabolic boost to your body.

Intermittent fasting helps you reduce your intake of calories and helps with weight loss. The primary reason why intermittent fasting is an effective weight loss technique is because it reduces your calorie intake. As such there is no calorie restrictions prescribed by this diet. All the different methods of intermittent fasting involve foregoing meals during the periods of fast. Unless you try to compensate for all this by eating more during the eating window, then you will certainly be consuming fewer calories than usual. Intermittent fasting can be a major contributor to weight loss if you carefully follow the protocols of this diet for at least three weeks. It isn't just fat loss that you will experience on this diet; you will also notice that you are losing fat from your abdominal region. The benefits of intermittent fasting are not restricted to just weight loss. This diet has a positive effect on your metabolic health and helps prevent any chronic diseases.

You don't have to necessarily count calories while following any method of intermittent fasting, but you need to maintain a calorie deficit if you want to lose weight. Intermittent fasting helps reduce your calorie intake without setting up any calorie restrictions.

One of the side effects of a diet that helps you lose fat is that it also causes you to burn muscle while burning fat. When it comes to intermittent fasting, you will not be burning any muscle mass and, in fact, it helps you gain lean muscle mass. The reduction in muscle mass while on intermittent fasting is quite low when compared to a diet that prescribes continuous calorie restriction.

Apart from this, it is also easier to eat healthily while following this diet. The simplicity of this diet is the main reason for all the benefits it offers. You can select any method of intermittent fasting and you will notice that you are eating healthier meals than before. If you want to follow the OMAD protocol, then you can eat only one meal per day. If you can eat only one meal, then you need to make sure that the meal that you eat will fill you up so that you can go through the day without feeling hungry. The foods that will fill you up for longer are foods rich in protein and fiber. So, knowingly or not you will start to incorporate healthy foods into your diet. For instance, eating a bowl of lettuce will make you feel fuller for longer than a packet of chips. So, you will be making healthier food choices.

Intermittent fasting is a wonderful dieting protocol that you can follow to lose weight. The main reason for weight loss on this diet is the reduction in the intake of calories.

So, by now, you know all that you must know about Intermittent Fasting and if you are willing to try this great lifestyle, I would be glad to make your life easier. In this very short section, I am going to give you some tips that you can use so you can deal with hunger and stick to your plan.

When I first started intermittent fasting it was like one year ago, I found about it from one of the best trainers out there in my opinion and it was one of the best things that I did to implement this in my life. I was not eating in the morning anyway, so it was easier for me to get started, but what really helped me out were his little tricks about making it easier, almost effortless to keep. One of the best things that you can do is to start drinking coffee and I mean black coffee without any sugar or milk. Why do you want to do this? Because black coffee is a great appetite suppressor, it helps you manage your hunger and for sure if you want to have a sensation of fullness you may want to drink it with sparkling water as well.

The last thing that I will mention is that it is easier to spend 4-8 hours after waking up without food. You can drink some cups of coffee with some water and this will help you manage your hunger much better.

Chapter 11:
Keto and Intermittent Fasting

Intermittent fasting and the Ketogenic diet are both hot topics that often fall into conversations these days, especially in the health and fitness industry. Some differences make you wonder if one is better than the other, or if they can both fit into your life.

Let's now compare intermittent fasting and the Ketogenic diet. We've already covered what each one does in the previous chapters, so let's see some brief similarities and differences that they share. Afterward, we will discuss some important tips on how to intermittent fast on the Ketogenic diet.

Similarities

Ketosis is a direct result of starving the body of either carbs or food in general. Therefore, the Ketogenic diet and intermittent fasting have much of the same benefits. They work with each other very well as they are aiming towards the same goal, entering and maintaining ketosis.

Just like the Ketogenic diet, intermittent fasting involves times of starving the body of either carbs or food. However, because you are still eating food on the Ketogenic diet, intermittent fasting gets the body into ketosis faster, because you're having no carbs or food at all when you're in the fasting state.

If you look at intermittent fasting and the Ketogenic diet, you can see that each one complements the other. Both have benefits for weight loss and health, and that has more to do with fasting than ketosis.

Differences
The most obvious and main difference is, one involves eating while the other doesn't. You can eat throughout the day and stay in ketosis when doing the Ketogenic diet. Whereas intermittent fasting means you won't eat any food for a certain amount of time.

The Ketogenic diet's goal is to put your body into ketosis. Intermittent fasting isn't a diet and just because you choose to do it, doesn't mean your goal is to be in ketosis. Some intermittent fast just to eat less during the day and to keep from overeating at night. Somebody might choose to do a Keto diet for more than just to lose weight.

Trying to Intermittent Fast on The Ketogenic Diet
- Don't try to intermittent fast in the first two weeks of starting the Ketogenic diet or if you follow the Standard American Diet. This is extremely important. Your body requires to get adapted to the Keto diet before you try intermittent fasting. Your body

must get used to eating low carbs so your body can utilize ketones for energy instead of using glucose. If you try intermittent fasting at the same time you begin the Keto diet, you will not succeed. You will be too glucose-dependent and too hungry to stick with it. There is some misinformation around about intermittent fasting. Intermittent fasting needs to be natural and not a struggle, and you should never feel hungry. It will be a gradual process and take time before it is used effectively.

- Don't try to plan intermittent fasting too much. You must listen to your body. Intermittent fasting works best if it is done naturally. If you realize its lunchtime, but you don't feel hungry, just skip it and eat at dinner time. If it is too late to eat? Skip dinner and eat breakfast. Most individuals are at ease to skip breakfast anyway. Try to eat about 1 pm and eat again about four hours before you go to bed, so your body has time to digest your foods.

- Start slow. Don't force yourself to do the complete intermittent fasting schedule immediately. You should never deprive or restrict yourself. When your body has become fat-adapted, you won't feel as hungry. Begin by staying away from snacks between meals. Next, try skipping regular meals. Do this only if you don't feel hungry.

- Stay busy. You might find it easier to skip meals if you are busy and don't spend time in the kitchen. You might be tempted to have a snack if you are around food, even if you don't feel hungry. It is easy to go without food when you are out shopping. Remember to drink plenty of liquid. Water, tea, or coffee is all you need.

Intermittent fasting is just one tool to help you reach your goal. It helps with weight loss, longevity, and many other things, but it is just one factor that helps you meet your target. Exercise, micronutrients, macronutrients, enough sleep, and stress levels are some things to consider. Never use intermittent fasting as a quick fix when you have overindulged.

Butter or bulletproof coffee will break your fasting. Eating coconut oil or butter will not keep you in a fasted state. Anything that has calories will have the same effect. That's why it is called fasting. If you must have coffee in the mornings, add some cream but skip the sugar, butter, and oils.

Remember as I mentioned earlier, intermittent fasting isn't for everyone. If you come under any of the conditions below you should not do intermittent fasting:

- Type 1 diabetes

- Type 2 diabetics should only do it under a doctor's supervision since they might need to adjust their medication.

- Bulimia nervosa

- Anorexia nervosa

- Adrenal or chronic fatigue disorders

- Breastfeeding

- Pregnant women

- Very stressed

- Exercise too much

- Don't get enough sleep

If you experience any side effects such as hormone imbalance, irregular periods, anxiety, or sleeplessness, you should consult your health care practitioner before continuing.

Chapter 12:
Intermittent Fasting Regiments

You also need to understand everything you can about what intermittent fasting does to your body, your mind, and your life. When you understand the kind of lifestyle you are getting into and the benefits you stand to gain, then you will be able to persevere and eventually practice intermittent fasting happily and diligently. Some of the protocols you may want to look at include;

- Eat-stop-eat protocol

- The 16-8 protocol

- The 5:2 fast diet

- The alternate day fasting

- One meal a day (OMAD)

16:8 Method

The 16:8 method (16 hours OFF and 8 hours ON) of Intermittent Fasting is the easiest and least hunger-inducing version of IF to integrate into your life. It is also known as the daily window fasting. This method works on its own, or as a stepping-stone towards longer fasts.

To practice 16:8 IF, you simply fast for 16 hours in a day, then eat for an 8-hour window. This is the shortest fast and the longest feasting window of any of the forms of intermittent fasting. When you follow 16:8 fasting method, you eat within the 8-hour window (maybe, 11 a.m. – 7 p.m.) and then fast for the remaining 16 hours (7 p.m. until 11 a.m.). The fasting and eating window can vary depending on the individual.

Alternate Day Fasting

This fasting has several different versions. Some of them allow consumption of 500 calories during the fast to make things easy. Starting with a 24-hour fast may be difficult for a beginner like you. True fast lovers will enjoy fasting 24 hours once or twice a week.

Eat Stop Eat (24-Hour Fast)

With this method, you fast for 24-hours once or twice every week. To start fasting, you start the fast after Saturday night dinner and fast until Sunday night dinner. This will give you a full 24-hour fast. Also, you can try a breakfast to breakfast or lunch to lunch method. You can drink water, tea, coffee and other non-caloric beverages during the fast. To lose weight, you must eat a normal amount of food during your eating period. Meaning, you shouldn't try to compensate for your lost meals due to the fast. You can start with 16 hours fast and then gradually increase the time.

5:2 Diet

This diet is called the Fast Diet. The diet recommends that you eat as usual for 5 days of the week and then eat 500 to 600 calories (men 600 calories, women 500 calories) daily during the remaining 2 days.

The Warrior Diet (20/4)

The Warrior diet is a combination of exercise and fasting. You will need to follow your gut feeling when it comes to choosing the right diet. Avoid getting tempted by processed food or junk food. Don't get too rigid with the types of macronutrients and calories that need to be consumed during the eating window. Instead, as the name implies, eat like a warrior! Our prehistoric warriors had little food during the day and had their meal at night, i.e., little food in the day and more food at night. After 20 hours, you can eat whatever foods you want if it is within a four-hour eating window.

The Warrior diet is more to do with vigorous exercising (even during the fasting days) and controlled food-intake. You will need to exercise when your stomach is completely empty (preferably as soon as you wake up). You will have only one meal in a day. If you can adapt to this type of intermittent fasting, you will be able to burn more fat (into energy) and will get a lean physique without the need to count your calories.

Your exercise routine should be total body strength training – squats, pushups, pull-ups, high jumps, skipping and presses. You can also include high-intensity cardio exercises, such as frog jumps or sprints, in between these sessions. These sessions can last for between 20 and 45 minutes.

Make sure you have a healthy organic, wholesome meal during your eating window. Add more vegetables, spices, greens and fruit to your plate. Drink enough water after your meal.

One Meal a Day Diet

The popularity of intermittent fasting is increasing every day. One method of IF that is steadily becoming quite popular is the One Meal a Day diet also known as the OMAD diet. Abstaining from food helps modulate your body's performance and when you fast for prolonged periods, it has a positive effect on your body and mind.

The OMAD protocol is designed in such a manner that the fasting ratio you need to follow is 23:1. It means that your body will be effectively fasting for 23 hours and the eating window is restricted to one hour. If you want to burn fat, trigger weight loss, improve your mental clarity and reduce the time that you spend on food, then eating one meal a day is a brilliant idea.

The OMAD method oscillates between periods of eating and fasting. This method of fasting reduces the eating window more than the other diets. While following this dieting protocol, you need to make sure that you consume your daily calories within one meal, and you fast for the rest of the day. OMAD helps you reap all the benefits of intermittent fasting and it simplifies your schedule as well. The ideal time to break your fast is between 4 and 7 p.m. When you do this, you give your body enough time to start digesting the food that you eat before you sleep.

From the perspective of evolution, humans aren't designed to eat three meals per day. As mentioned earlier, our ancestors' bodies were used to functioning optimally even when there was food scarcity. Intermittent fasting protocols like the OMAD tend to kickstart various cell functions in your body that are helpful to improve your overall health. It can be a challenge starting out with this method of dieting. There are three simple tips that you can follow to make the transition easier on yourself.

The first thing that you need to do is slowly cut back on the carbs that you consume. If you want to optimize the results of this diet and want the least amount of crankiness, then you must limit your carb intake. Your body tends to create a stock of glycogen in the body when lots of carbs are taken in. If there is always some glucose present in your body, then your body will not be able to shift into ketosis. Ketosis is essential to kickstart the process of burning fats. So, if you are trying to start this diet, then it is a good idea to start by slowly cutting back on your carb intake.

You need to ease your body into getting used to this fasting protocol. It can be quite difficult to go from eating three meals a day to just one meal a day. You need to ease the transition so that it doesn't feel like you are suffering. A simple way in which you can do this is by slowly getting your body used to the idea of eating fewer meals. So, if you are used to eating three meals per day and tend to snack in between the meals, then the first step is to eliminate all the snacks. Then you make gradual increments to the time between the meals and cut down on the number of meals you eat. If you do this, it will be quite easy to follow this diet.

Another simple way in which you can make this diet easier on your body is to consume some caffeine. A morning cup of coffee (devoid of milk and sugar) will make you feel fuller for longer and will keep your hunger pangs at bay. You will learn more about the different tips that you can follow to manage your hunger in the coming chapters.

Chapter 13:
Beginners 4 Week Plan

To start the Keto lifestyle is simple; many health and fitness "experts" make the Keto diet complicated. Here are the key points to getting started the right way with the Keto diet.

- You can eat generous servings of any type of meat, don't trim the fat off.

- You can eat all the vegetables you wish, just watch the carb count on veggies such as broccoli.

- You can have salads with most dressings.

- You can eat most cheeses.

- Use mayonnaise and olive oil on everything.

- Keep deviled eggs ready for yourself as a snack.

- Get creative with your meal choices; if it's an omelet, make it a bacon, cheddar, diced tomato and mushroom omelet.

- Eat when you're hungry not by a schedule.

- Drink lots of water to get rid of impurities in the body and to stave off constipation.

If you have a craving and binge on ice cream or cookies, don't worry just go right back on the diet after that last meal. You can have all the coffee and tea you want if add-ons such as milk, sugar, syrup and the like don't take you over your set carb count. Stay away from most sugary foods for the first 6 days, such as honey, jelly, syrups, cake, rice, cereals. Sunday go all out on whatever you like.

A Word on Cheating

If you must have that bagel or bowl of rice during the first week, go for it; don't beat yourself up over it. I want you to feel freedom over food not feel like a victim. And the same goes for if you lost all the weight you wanted and fell off and ate the wrong foods, no big deal. When following the Keto diet, there are things that you should consider:

1. This diet is not for everyone. Those who are undergoing medical attention such as cardiovascular diseases, gallbladder, diabetes, and pregnant women are discouraged from following this diet.

2. The Ketogenic diet should not be combined with other diets. Doing so could only compromise your health. Therefore, choose which diet really works for you. Before starting with a new one, allow your body to rest and adjust for at least 2 weeks.

3. Consult with your nutritionist. Ask a nutritionist to supervise your progress even if you are at your fittest. If you are into strength training, it is more important to consult a nutritionist. This kind of diet requires careful meal planning as it is easy to slip and go back to your usual eating habit especially when you find the diet uncomfortable and maintaining it becomes a bit of a challenge.

4. Drink plenty of water. If there is one major drawback of the Keto diet, that would have to be constipation. Since water is flushed out from the body quickly, there is usually a delay in bowel movement. Therefore, drinking plenty of water along with consuming food rich in fiber is important while on the Ketogenic Diet.

You're ready to go shopping. It can be an overwhelming task at first, so here are some helpful tips to keep you on track. Plan your meals ahead before heading to the grocery or store. Write all your ingredients and know what you need and what you already have. Do your purchases on a seasonal basis and note when there is abundance of fresh produce? Some of the items to purchase:

- Keto meats – steaks, ground beef, shrimp, pork chops, bacon, salmon

- Keto vegetables – broccoli, kale, cucumber, asparagus, spinach, peppers, cauliflower, mushrooms, squash

- Keto fruits – almost all berries

- Dairy products – half and half, butter, most cheese like Parmesan, cream, Swiss, blue, shredded cheddar

- Other Keto pantry items – almonds, hazelnuts, cocoa powder, macadamia, sunflower seeds, olives, all the spices, coconut oil

Always buy the items in bulk. This is a wonderful way of saving money. Be ready to buy when there are offers or coupons before they expire.

Start with the Keto Diet First

By starting with the Keto Diet first, it will help you transition your body into a ketosis state, so you begin to burn excess fat for energy to facilitate weight loss. By consuming low glycemic fruits and leafy green vegetables, moderate high-quality protein and significant healthy fats will increase your satiety and help you feel full.

However, minimize and eliminate all processed foods wherever possible including sugar. While this may be difficult initially (I know as I was in the same place), you will see benefits much quicker. This sets up well to integrate Intermittent Fasting next with your Keto Diet as your body will be already accustomed to being in a fat burning state.

Integrate Intermittent Fasting Next

Intermittent Fasting promotes weight loss as well, improves your key physiology functions and detoxifies your body. You can amplify these benefits when you combine Intermittent Fasting with the Keto Diet.

Select your fasting protocol. The most popular method of Intermittent Fasting is a time restricted feeding (TRF) protocol as discussed earlier called 16/8. This means you don't eat for 16 hours and consume your meals within an eight (8) hour window. The 16/8 protocol will be the easiest to start with since it's close to what you normally do. You can then transition to longer periods of fasting as your body adjusts to fasting on a regular basis.

As you fast, your body reaches into its stores of glycogen to provide energy to your body. Once your glycogen stores are depleted, your body will begin to burn stored fat to provide energy once ketosis begins. Fasting assists the body to enter ketosis since there is no other source of energy available during the fasting period.

Break Your Fast with Keto-Friendly Wholesome Foods

The next step is to eat Keto-friendly foods when you break your fast. For instance, if you're eating window stretches from noon until 8 pm at night then the food that you can consume during this period must be Keto-friendly. Use the Keto food list to make sure that you always have Keto ingredients and supplies in your pantry. Go through the various recipes given in this book to cook tasty and healthy food.

You may also experiment a little before getting the perfect combination of the various Intermittent Fasting protocols, the Keto Diet and your personal lifestyle.

Always consult your physician before you start the Keto Diet and any of the Intermittent Fasting protocols.

The goal of the transitional phase on the Keto diet is to allow you to ease into your new lifestyle. While it is certainly possible to jump right into a new lifestyle, it is not the easiest or most encouraging approach. We are all struggling with enough difficulties in life already. There is no need to challenge yourself to do a one-eighty lifestyle shift when instead you can ease into confidently over the span of four weeks.

There's some stuff you need to do as preparation for the Keto Diet journey to come! It helps to have all your helpful tools assembled before you begin, so that you're fully prepped and ready to go. That includes purchasing a Keto Blood or Breath monitor, buying the necessary cooking implements and kitchen tools for making Keto meals, and investing in a new notebook as your food diary. You'll also want to go online and find a Macro calculator. Fill out the questionnaire and then write the results here:

- Fats: _____ grams

- Proteins: _____ grams

- Carbohydrates: _____ grams

- Total Calories: _____

It's also helpful to set goals. How much weight are you intending to lose by the end of these four weeks? Do you have any other Keto Diet goals? Add those to your food diary to help you stay on track.

- Weight Loss goal: _____ pounds in _____ weeks

- Fitness goal: _____

You may also want to come up with a meal plan for your first week. Include the recipes that you'll need, too. You'll also want to purchase the ingredients for at least the first seven days of Keto meals, based on your personalized Macros.

You'll notice in Week One there's no exercise plan (yet). That's because we want your body to get used to Intermittent Fasting before we add exercise to it. Let's just focus on your eating plan and eating schedule. There's plenty of time to add exercise later!

Whew! There's a lot to do before Day 1, but these are all the foundational tools you'll need to get through your first week, both Keto dieting and Intermittent Fasting. Now you're ready to start and you've laid the groundwork for a successful first month!

Week One

Day 1

Day 1 is going to be a normal, regular day without any major changes to your Ketogenic Diet at all. We're going to ease slowly into Intermittent Fasting. So, for today all you've got to do is cook and eat three regular Keto meals plus a snack/dessert/drink. Follow your own customized meal plan. You can also eat your meals whenever you want. Make sure you reach your Macros. Track what you ate in your food diary. Monitor either your breath or blood and check for ketosis.

There are no specific guidelines about exactly when you should measure ketone levels. In the morning, ketone concentrations are lower and higher in the evening. Two factors throw off ketone levels: right after exercising and when you're dehydrated.

Going forward, just monitor your ketones at a consistent time every time you do. If you test at 10:00 am today on Day 1, then always test at 10:00 am on future days. You're trying to find your baseline and your normal readings. Then, when it changes, you'll know!

Day 2

Today is your first attempt at Intermittent Fasting! We're going to do a skipped meal. Many Keto Dieters skip breakfast, because that's an easy meal to skip. A lot of us just aren't hungry in the mornings. Also, skipping breakfast extends your fast from the night before, increasing its benefits. You can skip lunch or skip dinner, too.

Whichever meal you decide to skip, make sure for the remainder of your meals, you're getting in your Macros. This means having extra Macro grams at the other meals than you normally would. How did this first day of fasting go? Were you hungry during the skipped meal period? Or, was it relatively easy? Record your experience.

Day 3

If Day 2 went well by both fasting and adding Macros to other meals, you're welcome to repeat it on Day 3. Pick a meal to skip and increase your Macros for the other meals.

If Day 2 was difficult and you were very hungry between meals, then just go back to a regular eating schedule on the Keto Diet. Cook and eat your three Ketogenic meals just like you normally would.

Day 4

Repeat Day 3. Skip one of your meals as your time spent Intermittent Fasting and eat your other meals with the increased Macro grams. Check to see that you're in ketosis using a monitoring tool. Track your Macros, your calories, and your Keto monitoring readout in a food diary.

Day 5

No Intermittent Fasting today. You are going to cook and eat your Keto meals as normal, with the Macros spread throughout the day. This gives your body a chance to rest between times of fasting. You may find as you proceed that you become more fat-adapted, which will slowly decrease your hunger. For those of you who like tracking data, you can check your ketones again today. Staying consistently in ketosis will help you lose the weight, too.

Day 6

Today, you'll practice Intermittent Fasting for a longer period. You're going to have an eating window of 10 hours, with 14 hours off for fasting. This eating window can start at any time in the morning and continue for the ten hours. For example, you could start it at 8:00 am and continue until 6:00 pm. After your eating window is done, you're not to eat any solid foods or broths until tomorrow. You can drink some water with lemon slices to keep up your electrolytes.

During your 10-hour eating window is when you'll consume all your Macros. You can split up the Macros into any meal combination you like. A heavy breakfast, light lunch, and heavy dinner would be an option. Or a combination that fits you. Don't forget to snack within those ten hours, so you can reach your Macro counts. Track everything in your food diary too.

Day 7

Yay, you've got to the end of your first week! Celebrate by weighing yourself. Have you lost any weight yet? A healthy weight loss schedule is up to two pounds per week. How are your energy levels? Are you doing well with the Intermittent Fasting times? Did you prefer the skipped meals or the 10-hour window? Tweak and adjust as the schedule go forward.

Today, you'll want to repeat Day 6 by doing another 10-hour window. It must be the exact same time as yesterday, to make sure you're getting the full fourteen-hour fasting cycle. So, if you started your ten-hour window at 8:00 am yesterday, you'll start it at 8:00 am today. Again, get all your Macros in your eating window. When it stops, that's when it's time to fast.

Week Two

Day 8

After several days of skipped meals and two days of 10-hour eating windows, it's time to shorten you're eating window and increase your fasting time. What time did your 10-hour eating window end yesterday? Count forward sixteen hours, and that's when your 8-hour eating window should start today. For example, if you ended your 10-hour window at 6:00 pm last night, you'll start your 8-hour eating window at 10:00 am today, and it will end at 6:00 pm. That's sixteen hours of fasting, consuming nothing but water with lemon slices for electrolytes. You'll want to eat all your Macros in your shorter 8-hour window. That includes breakfast, lunch, dinner, and your snack/dessert/drink.

Day 8 is also a good time to plan out meals for Week Two. Find recipes for those meals with the included Macros and go shopping for your ingredients to restock your kitchen. Also, monitor your ketones again. Are you staying in ketosis? If so, great! If not, adjust your Macros, follow the troubleshooting tips in the previous chapter, and get back into ketosis.

Day 9

The 8-hour feeding window from yesterday is repeated today, at the exact same time you started it yesterday. Eat all your Macros in the 8 hours. If you're having a bit of a challenge consuming enough of your Fat Macros in a shorter time frame, try taking some MCT oil. Start with a small amount, like a teaspoon, since it does cause nausea in some people. A 1 Tablespoon serving has 100 calories and 14 grams of good fats.

Day 10

Repeat your 16-hour Intermittent Fasting/8-hour Keto Dieting routine today as well. Just make sure you're consuming all your daily Macros in those 8 hours. If you're having difficulty, it's okay to go back to a regular Keto eating schedule. Adjust the eating window time, too, if it's not working out. If it is working out, great! After trying to fast for ten days, your body does start to change.

Day 11

Today is the day to not only continue your 16-hour fasting/8-hour eating plan, but to try incorporating some exercise into it. You don't have to, but getting exercise is wonderful for your body and has so many benefits. You'll sleep better, too. Since your body is adjusting to a fasting schedule, don't overdo it on your workouts. A gentle 30-minute routine to get your heart rate up is usually all it takes. Just like yesterday, eat your Macros within the 8 hours. Track and record your experience.

Day 12

Today, we're going to shorten our eating window by one more hour, thus increasing our fasting window. You'll now be fasting for 17 hours and eating for 7 hours, and we'll repeat that cycle for several days. When was the end of yesterday's eating window? Count forward 17 hours, and that's when your 7-hour time frame begins. Now, you'll be eating all your Macros in a 7-hour period. Take your mineral supplements and gently increase your MCT oil dosage as well. Get plenty of water during fasting periods. You can add 30 minutes of exercise, but not if you are feeling weak or struggling with this eating routine. Give your body time to adjust.

Day 13

How did yesterday go when eating for just 7 hours during the day? The time goes by quick! By now, you should be able to tell when you're staying in ketosis even during those fasting times. It's noticeable! You'll feel it if you knock yourself out.

Repeat your 7-hour eating window schedule from yesterday. You can add exercise, too. Eat and track your Macros, making sure you're also getting your recommended calories. As eating windows get shorter, many Keto Dieters reduce the number of meals to two, plus a snack or Keto beverage. Eating twice a day works out for a lot of people, so give it a try!

Day 14

Congrats – you've reached the end of the second week. You went from a 10-hour window down to a 7-hour eating window, increasing your fasting time by three hours! That's three extra hours your body is spending pulling fuel sources from existing fat cells rather than relying on incoming fuel sources from your meals. You also added exercise, which burns even more fat in your cells. You've started to supercharge the Keto Diet effects by fasting.

It's time to assess the week. How did you do on your increased Intermittent Fasting? Was it easy to add exercise to it? Have you been tracking your Fats, Proteins, and Carbohydrates each day?

Weigh yourself to see if you've lost more weight. If so, excellent! If not, then you need to undertake some troubleshooting tips to help you. In addition to sticking to your 7-hour eating window today, check your ketones again using your monitor. Intermittent Fasting helps bump you into ketosis faster than simply cutting carbs. So, that's a noticeable change this week.

Week Three

Day 15

Day 15 begins with a new eating plan for this week, but now it's going to be based on a new eating window of just 6 hours. That's 18 hours spent fasting the rest of the time. Count forward from yesterday one additional hour, and that's when your fast should begin. You can adjust and tweak your fasting schedule during Days 15 and 16 to see which the best 6-hour timeframe for you is. But by Day 17, your routine should be consistent. Consistency with your feeding/fasting cycles is key to getting all the benefits from doing this.

You're also going to do your first 24-hour fast this week, so plan for that in your schedule. Go shopping for your Keto Diet ingredients and restock your cupboards. Make sure you have plenty of mineral rich foods for the day after your fast and keep a good supply of salty broths on hand, too.

Day 16

Today is the second day of your new 6-hour eating window and 18-hour fast. Eat all your Macros inside of those 6 hours and track them in your food diary. Are you feeling more energy? Many Keto Dieters enjoy such a short eating window, since it really makes the effects of fasting noticeable. You can add some exercise to your schedule as well. Start with 30 minutes and gradually increase, depending on your fitness goals and how well you're doing on your fasting/feeding cycles. It's okay to cut back on your fitness if you're feeling weak or sluggish in any way.

Day 17

Continue with your 6-hour feeding/18-hour fasting schedule today. Get in as many Macros as you can within those short six hours. Add your exercise to your routine, too. Make any adjustments like necessary. During fasting times, you should only be drinking water with a bit of lemon for electrolytes.

Day 18

Today is all about preparing for tomorrow's 24-hour fast. It's imperative that you eat all your Macros in their 6-hour feeding window today. Abstain from exercising, to give your muscles a chance to fully rest today and tomorrow. Check that you're in ketosis, too. If you're not, don't do the fast. Try a few more days of 18-hour fasts before you attempt a longer one. Once you're in ketosis, you can do a 24-hour fast.

Day 19

Today is your first 24-hour Intermittent Fasting day! Count 24 hours from the beginning of yesterday's fasting time and don't eat anything during that whole time. For example, if your 6-hour eating window ended at 6:00 pm yesterday, you're not to eat anything until 6:00 pm today.

Break your fast gently with some MCT oil and eat mineral rich foods like salmon, dark greens, avocado, nuts, and olives. Don't worry about getting in all your Macros but do stop all eating at least two hours before bedtime. Abstain from exercise today, too.

Day 20

Time to return to your 6-hour feeding/18-hour fasting cycle. How did yesterday's extended fast go? Make sure to rehydrate yourself today with plenty of water. Today, you do want to eat all your Macros just like you did on Day 18, even if you're not hungry. You're helping your body refuel itself with good fats. If you want to return to your exercise routine, you can if you feel up to it. Don't overdo it, though!

Day 21

Day 19's extended 24-hour fasting time was quite a challenge, but you got through it and did great! That's cause for celebration, and you can weigh yourself again, too. How close are you to meeting the weight loss goals you set before your monthly challenge began? If you've lost at least 5 pounds, then it's a good idea to go back to an online Macro calculator. Recalculate your Macros considering your new weight.

How is the 6-hour eating window going for you? If you prefer the 7-hour or the 8-hour timeframes, it's perfectly fine to return to those schedules instead! The important thing is to stay in ketosis. Check it again today using the Breath or Blood Monitor.

Week Four

Day 22

This week has an advanced 48-hour multi-day fasting time period that takes up Days 24 and Day 25. You're welcome to try it! Many of you have already experienced extraordinary health benefits just by doing the Intermittent Fasting so far, and we know you love a challenge! If at any point, you're feeling overwhelmed or sick or not enjoying the process in any way, it's okay to return to a normal Keto Diet schedule.

This is the beginning of the week, so it's a good idea to plan out your meals, shop for the ingredients, and stock your kitchen in preparation. Remember to purchase the mineral supplements and mineral-rich foods you'll need on Day 26 to break your fast. As for today, just continue your 6-hour eating window like you did yesterday.

Day 23

Today is about preparing for your multi-day fast, which begins tomorrow. Eat all your Macros within your 6-hour window, tracking them to make sure you've eaten enough good fats. Take note of the time your 6-hour window ends. You'll count 48 hours in advance, and that's when you can break your fast. Abstain from exercising today and throughout the fast as well. You can take light walks, but just don't be too strenuous on yourself.

Day 24

Fast all day today! Drink water take a mineral supplement and satisfy any hunger pangs with a small teaspoon of MCT oil. It's 100% good fats, and it won't affect either you are being in ketosis or take away the benefits of the fast.

Day 25

Fast all day today as well. Drink water take another mineral supplement, and you can have another teaspoon of MCT oil during the fast. Fast until it's been 48 hours since your Day 23 eating window ended. Break your fast with a low carb meal that includes mineral-rich foods like salmon, dark greens, and avocado. Don't try to get in your complete Macros before bedtime.

Day 26

Ease back into your 18-hour fast/6-hour eating window today. Eat your full Macros during those six hours. How did your 48-hour fast go? You can check your ketones to see how well you did! For most of you, staying in ketosis while fasting has really boosted its benefits!

Day 27

Repeat Day 26 with your normal 6-hour eating window. Today, though, you've given your body enough of a chance to rest from the effects of the 48-hour fast. So, you can add back in your regular exercise routine. Eat and track your Macros.

Day 28

Many congrats to you for getting through an amazing month of Keto Dieting and Intermittent Fasting! You can weigh yourself again and enjoy the results from your hard work. Go back to your food diary that you've been keeping throughout this month-long journey. Was it easier than you expected or more difficult? What was your personal experience with Intermittent Fasting? Casual 'fasters might want to stick with the skipped meals. More advanced 'fasters' really like the shorter eating windows. Those advanced 'fasters' looking to drop either their weight quickly or reach fitness goals quickly would do well to stay on shorter eating windows and incorporate longer fasts at least once a month.

However, your experience went, you deserve to celebrate! Show off your progress by posting "before" and "after" pictures of yourself.

Chapter 14:
Big No No's

Foods to Avoid: these foods are strictly out of bounds.

- All grains: wheat, oats, rye, quinoa, cereals, bread, millets, buck-wheat, barley, corn

- Starchy vegetables: potatoes, yams, sweet potatoes

- Most fruits: bananas, apples, papayas, grapes, citrus, pears, peaches, pineapple, mangoes, nectarines

- Sugar: maple syrup, honey, basically anything with sugar

- Juice: all kinds as most juices come from sugary fruits

- Beans and legumes: this include all beans, chickpeas and lentils

- Alcohol: most alcoholic drinks have lots of sugar, so they are a big no-no (small amounts of dry wine in cooking is okay)

- Condiments and sauces: most bought sauces are high in sugars and carbs, so it's best to make your own out of simple, whole ingredients such as olive oil and vinegar.

Common Mistakes

With everything said and done, it should be mentioned that there are some common mistakes that are made by new Keto enthusiasts.

- Since no proper definition of how much carb is actually "Low-Carb" exists, some people often tend to shoot their carb intake to a very high level while still considering that they are under "Low-Carb." The level of daily carb should be around 20-50 for an optimal experience, but a maximum of 100-150g.

- It is understood that as a macronutrient, protein is very important as a bodybuilding food. It improves the level of satiety and encourages fat burning. Yet, be aware of having too much protein as the excess might turn into glucose, which will once more be burned up for energy instead of fat.

- A very big mistake made by newcomers is they naturally think that lowering the level of fat alongside the carbs might increase the fat loss. That is wrong! Keep in mind that you need the fat in your body if you want to encourage the burning of fat!

- When on Keto, you need to reduce the level of insulin. While on a Ketogenic diet, your insulin levels will go down significantly, which helps greatly to relieve the level of bloat. Still, with that very process, electrolytes from our body are also flushed away. Therefore, balance the decrease in electrolytes by having a good amount of sodium (salt) intake to make sure that your kidneys are safe, and you don't have problems such as fatigue, constipation or a light headache.

Mistake #1: Hidden Carbs

Not counting hidden carbohydrates is one of the most common mistakes committed while on Ketogenic diet. First, food manufacturers are not completely accurate with the amount of carbohydrates on their labels. Read ingredients on the packaged food and make sure there are not any ingredients on there that would account for some extra carbohydrates. Those hidden carbs can add up fast.

The second way this can happen is when you look at the ingredients and see that there are carbohydrates, but you fail to look at the serving size. For example, some candies and candy bars are listed as two servings, meaning you need to double the amount of carbohydrates on the package if you plan on eating the entire thing!

Mistake #2: Sweeteners and Fruit

Fruit contains a ton of excess carbohydrates in the form of fructose, especially when it's completely ripened. Limit your fruit consumption or you will go over your carb limit very quickly.

Mistake #3: Too Much Protein

In excess, protein can convert into glucose via gluconeogenesis. You want to burn ketones, not glucose. Ketogenic diet, protein makes up approximately 25% of your calories.

Mistake #4: Not Eating Enough!

If you are not eating enough, and severely restrict your calories, you will feel hungry. You will likely get irritable, and the diet won't last. For lasting results, stick to the 70% fats, 25% protein, 5% carbs. You'll be eating a lot fatter than on a normal diet, this might take some adjustment.

Mistake #5: Not Enough Sodium

Get salty. During ketosis, insulin levels reduce greatly. Lowered insulin triggers the kidneys to dump sodium. Increase sodium intake to avoid deficiency. Sea salt is healthiest.

The only thing left now is to know what you need and going to do, to prepare yourself for the journey ahead.

Chapter 15:
Tips and Tricks and FAQs

There are important considerations you need to know before you embark on the Ketogenic diet. Below are some important tips to recap and help you be successful with this diet.

Tip #1: Count Carbohydrates

There are some useful apps out there you can find on your phone or online calculators to count net carbohydrates. However, there is a simple way to do this. When in doubt, simply take the total carbohydrates listed on a product's label and subtract the fiber from that total amount. This is your net carbohydrates. Of course, if you're eating fresh, whole foods, this is a little more difficult because there isn't any label packaging. That's where apps are handy.

Tip #2: Planning and Preparation

Planning for this diet, you need to shop for the right foods and cook at home more. Creating and following a meal plan is key to success. Sit down and outline your day/week/month, and don't forget to plan for snacks!

Tip #3: Eat Enough Fat

With this diet, fat makes up 70% of your caloric intake. That's a lot of fat. In order to get enough calories, stock up on the fat. Even if you are in a calorie deficit, you're still eating 70% fat. If you're having trouble getting enough fat, stock up on the olive oil, coconut oil and butter. You'll be eating a lot of these fats, bulk purchase to save money.

Tip #4: Make Keto A Lifestyle

It's a good idea to try turning the Ketogenic diet into a lifestyle plan. This means making the diet into a habit. In order to do this, you should first try not to overwhelm yourself and don't get upset if you back-pedal and don't follow the plan. Immediately return to it and try again.

Commitment is key! Commit to the Ketogenic diet for a week, two weeks, and then maybe a month. By the end of a month, it will turn into a habit and living this new lifestyle won't seem as difficult.

Tip #5: Drink Plenty of Water

Entering a stage of ketosis will naturally deplete your body's water supply. Therefore, you need to drink tons of water in order to stay hydrated, but not only that, you need to keep an eye on your electro-lyte levels too.

Tip #6: Increase Salt Intake

As levels of insulin circulating through your body lower, your kidneys will begin excreting some excess sodium. Eat more salt to avoid electrolyte deficiency.

Tip #7: Experiment
Have fun with this diet! Although there are restrictions, compared to most diets, it's flexible and so delicious. Play around with recipes and different ingredients. Enjoy trying new foods you might have never explored, just make sure you're following your macros.

Tip #8: Keto + Intermittent Fasting
A common practice for rapid weight loss is combining Ketogenic diet with intermittent fasting. This is common as many people find it easier and more convenient to meet their macros with this pattern of eating. Intermittent fasting is a pattern of eating in which you cycle between periods of fasting (fasted state) and eating (fed state).

Tip #9: Patience
Be patient. Follow the diet, and the results will show over time. Don't stress out if results don't show up immediately. Good things come to those who are disciplined and have patience. Eating more carbs will be tempting, if you really want the results, stick to your macros.

- Cook for yourself – freeze the remaining servings or save half of the recipes, if needed.

- Swap your meals – you can swap your meals any time of the day. Eat breakfast for lunch or lunch for dinner. Your meal plan depends on you!

- Try to skip the snacks – while you should feel satisfied with the 3 main meals, keep Keto-friendly snacks close by.

- Only eat when hungry – if you don't feel hunger, don't eat.

- Substitute – fish, pork, and lamb can be substituted for one another in recipes due to their similar nutritional value.

Understand that diet plans are not suitable for everyone: Make sure that your daily requirements match your recipes and diet plan. Make small adjustments and reduce the portions if needed. Don't worry if you go over your protein intake a bit, as it will not kick you out of ketosis and will keep hunger at bay. If you find yourself lacking enough fat in your diet, add more fat by adding oils and fatty foods according to your adjustments.

Tips for Going Out

The Ketogenic diet can seem easy enough for the times when you are cooking your own food at home, but it can be quite a challenge to eat out at dining establishments or social events if you are not prepared. When going to a restaurant, call ahead or look at the menu before you arrive and see what they have. Keep an eye out for grilled or steamed vegetables and see if they can poach an egg if you need some extra protein. Otherwise, have a snack before you go out and simply order a vegetable side. If you can find a restaurant that serves breakfast items all day, you are all set! Just be sure to stay away from industrial oils like canola, and always ask they your food be prepared with pure olive oil or butter.

Often the salad dressings served in restaurants are loaded with unhealthy oils and sugar. If you believe that you may be enjoying a side of vegetables or a salad as your entrée, ask if they can provide you with a lemon and some pure extra virgin olive oil to use as a dressing along with some salt and black pepper. Otherwise, you could sneak in a small bottle of extra virgin olive oil just in case they do not have any of their own to serve. Keep in mind that many restaurants serve what they call an "olive oil blend," which is olive oil blended with canola oil. Most of the time, you can pretty much bet that what they are giving you is not pure unless you specifically ask, or even state that you have a severe allergy. This makes them more likely to take your request seriously.

When going to a social event, the best course of action is almost always to bring a dish. Choose something that is substantial enough to be eaten on its own, like a salad with plenty of nuts. If you happen to be in a dinner party where everything is to be prepared for you and you do not have the option to bring a dish of your own, have a chat with the host and explain to him or her that you have special dietary needs. If he or she will be cooking meat as the main dish, find out what sides are being prepared. If any of them are low in carbohydrates, perhaps imply that they could make an additional amount of that side so that you may enjoy it as your main course. You can always have a quick snack before you arrive, such as a hard-boiled egg or some nuts for protein and fat.

Tips for Staying Optimum Ketosis Level

1) Testing Ketone Levels – the most inexpensive way to do this is testing your urine for acetoacetate, the ketone measured in urine. The test can be carried out early in the morning or after dinner when on a Keto diet. You will just dip the ketone urine strips in your urine. The darker the strip the higher the ketone levels are and the better that it is. The shades can range from pink to purple.

2) Sustained and Ample Protein Consumption – the keyword here is ample which does not equate to excessive protein intake. The suggested formula to use is multiplying your body weight in pounds by 0.55 to 0.77; for example, your ideal weight is 140-lbs then your protein intake daily should be between 77g to 107.8g.

3) Go into a Fat Fast or Short Fast – this is going for fasts like an intermittent fasting. Example of a short fast is to go fasting for at least 14 hours in between dinner and your breakfast the next day to induce ketosis. Fat fasting on the other hand is just eating 1,000 calories in one day with the bulk of the food coming from fats. You can do this once or twice a week to induce ketosis.

4) Boost Your Intake of healthy Fats – since the Keto diet is composed mostly between 80%-90% fats, it is only sensible to consume the healthy types of fats and they are coconut oil, butter, avocado oil, olive oil, and the likes. And if you are on a Keto diet to lose weight, mind your calories too.

5) Increase your Physical Activity – studies show that when you are physically active, it increases your ketone levels. But, if you're still new to the Keto diet, it may take your body one to four weeks to adapt to this new metabolic pathway and hence physical performance can be temporarily reduced.

6) Add Coconut Oil in the Diet – coconut oil is a type of fat known as medium-chain triglycerides (MCTs) and studies have shown that this type of fat can create a more sustained level of ketosis.

7) Strictly Lower Carb Intake – Remember the first pathway that the body uses? By breaking down carbs into glucose and then using glucose as fuel for the bodily processes? That's what you completely need to avoid in order to get into a ketosis. It is suggested that if you want to lose weight fewer than 21 grams of carb consumption daily is the paramount goal.

Tips for Working Out While on Keto and IF

It's okay to exercise on an empty stomach: Many people believe exercising on an empty stomach reduces performance. They also believe exercising on an empty stomach will cause muscle loss and not the desired fat loss.

This is not true! You still have fat as an energy source. The only time your body starts to digest the proteins for fuel is when you aren't getting enough fat in your diet.

Another point worth mentioning is the type of exercise and diet. Muscle loss can occur with certain types of exercise, not based on whether you eat before exercising. Calorie restrictive diets or eating too little can contribute to muscle loss. You lose muscle not because you fasted before exercising but rather because you are generally not eating enough.

Too much cardio can also be a culprit in muscle loss. Many health and fitness experts recommend weightlifting over cardio to lose weight. This also helps tone the body while burning fats.

Exercises to perform while fasting or on ketogenesis: Some conditions promote muscle loss while excess fat is minimally burned. One is when you lose a lot of weight too fast within a short period. Another is when you eat too little but exercise a lot. Another is simply exercising too much with the wrong type of workout.

The intensity of the exercise is important when exercising in a Ketogenic state. You must aim to train with low intensity until your body is well adapted to the diet. High-intensity exercises for a long period require glucose, which you do not have in abundance during ketogenesis. Your body cannot produce ketones quickly enough to supply you with energy for long intense workouts. If you train during fasting periods, use low-intensity exercises. Steady-state, lower intensity cardio aerobic or cardio exercises work well.

Anaerobic exercise such as HIIT or weightlifting should be avoided until you are adapted and should not be done on fasting days. If you need, or want, to train with higher intensity during ketogenesis and find that your performance is limited by Keto, follow a targeted Keto diet. Eat fast-acting carbohydrate foods 30 minutes before a workout. One example is fruit. Limit the number of carbohydrates to 15 to 30 grams only. That will be enough to fuel your HIIT, especially if you do long HIIT workouts. I stick to 20-minute HIIT workouts and never need to add in carbs. Listen to your body and adjust as needed.

More Favorite Tips and Tricks

Plan Your Meals Smartly: Start your meal planning in advance and determine which foods you will need to prepare the meals for the whole week. Use your free time to prepare these foods in advance and store in refrigerator/freezer in containers. Similarly, make a list of food to purchase, go to grocery store and purchase ingredients for the whole week and store in your fridge and pantry.

Pick the Right Containers: Purchase containers according to your freezer size and your requirements. Always purchase containers that are BPA free and freezer safe. Similarly, buy bowls that are oven and microwave safe, so that you can re-heat the recipes in your bowl and serve them warm.

Use Frozen Vegetables: When it comes to preparing vegetables and fruits such as tomatoes, avocado, onions, cucumber, etc. Just chop them or make them as per recipe direction and store them in containers in the freezer. Frozen prepared vegetables save a lot of your time to prepare recipes as all you need to do is just to take them out from the freezer, thaw them and use directly to make recipes.

Store in Advance: For smoothies, you can place all the ingredients in fridge or freezer and blend them whenever you want to make smoothies. Similarly, you can prepare all your desserts in advance and store in the freezer. You can have them whenever you want. You can also prepare them in more quantity so that you can use them to serve on multiple days.

Be Patient to Master the Skill: Always remember that prepping meals requires some time to learn perfectly and will get better with experience. So, if you end up spoiling some ingredients, it's very normal. Try with simple recipes and try storing a few components first and then move up the ladder. Don't rush into learning everything at once.

Frequently Asked Questions

By now, you are aware of what is meant by Keto diet and intermittent fasting, and what you might expect from choosing to implement as your lifestyle. Here are some frequently asked questions to cover all relevant information. You can also use this section as a quick reference guide.

Q: How long will it take to get into ketosis?

The Ketogenic diet is not one that you can use intermittently, as you might with a fad diet. Its intention is not being a quick fix. As with any change that impacts our body, it takes a while to adjust and eventually reach the state of ketosis. It can take from 2 days to a whole week, give or take a little, considering your body, how much physical activity you are doing, and what you are (or aren't) eating. Some say that the fastest means of achieving ketosis is to do physical activity as much as possible on an empty stomach (like intermittent fasting), restricting your carb intake to no more than 20 grams a day, and maintaining proper hydration and electrolytes.

Q: Do I have to count calories?

Calories are going to matter at the end of the day. For weight loss, you need a calorie deficit and counting calories can be useful. However, it is time-consuming and tedious. Your job is to eat properly and never go too far into a deficit or too far over your limit. With the Ketogenic diet, you don't have to worry about calories as much because the fats and proteins fill you up and keep you feeling full for a longer period. However, if you exercise, you might want to be vigilant.

Q: Is it possible to eat too much fat?

Yes, it is possible to eat too much fat. In the end, you must be calorie deficit in order to lose weight. While most people are going to find it hard to overeat on a low carbohydrate high-fat diet, it is still possible to do. Calculate your macros and stick with those in order to lose weight. If your objective is maintaining your weight, or gain weight, you can eat even more fat.

Q: How much weight will I lose?

As with achieving ketosis, this is very individual. It depends not only on what you're eating (slightly more or fewer carbs or fat) and how much exercise you're getting but also just your genetic makeup. If you add a lot of exercise to your regimen, you will speed up and sometimes even increase your total amount of weight loss. You can also eliminate certain foods that may cause your weight loss to slow, like artificial sweeteners like Splenda (science suggests these actually can cause weight gain), wheat products or wheat-contaminated products (anything that may have trace amounts, especially if you might have an intolerance), dairy products, and low-fat processed foods. In the initial days or weeks, you may notice a very rapid weight loss. Unfortunately, this isn't fat, but rather, water loss. The Keto diet is a diuretic, which means you'll be having to urinate a lot more frequently, and it'll seem like you've lost a lot of weight, even though it's just water. On the upside, this means that your body is adjusting and likely heading towards ketosis, which is exactly what you want. It's in this state of ketosis that you'll really start burning off some fat.

Q: I started this diet, and now I don't feel good. What's going on?

As your body adjusts to this new state, it's very common for you to feel a bit under the weather and flu-like. Many people report experiencing headaches and some brain fogginess as well. Like mentioned before, ketosis causes a diuretic state, which means losing a lot of water from your body. With the drastic water loss and the consumption of our last remaining stores of glycogen, you're peeing out important electrolytes and you need to replace them ASAP. You need to be always hydrated by ensuring that you drink lots of water, and make sure to bump up your salt intake as well. Jerky, bacon, sausage, pepperoni, salted nuts, and even broths (both meat and veggie) are all excellent choices for getting the sodium you need. Replacing your electrolytes and staying properly hydrated will help lessen the "Keto flu" while your body adjusts. Remember to stay on top of these things even after being on the diet for a significant amount of time, as a drop-in electrolyte at any time will cause you to feel pretty icky.

Q: I have stopped losing weight, what's gone wrong and what can I do?

With any kind of new diet and exercise routine, weight loss plateaus happen, and the Ketogenic diet is no exception. There are various things that can cause this problem, but luckily there are also several things that you can try to help you get around this rut. You can try intermittent fasting, changing your workout routine, tweaking your diet - or all these things if you're really looking to shatter the plateaus. Try out the following in the given to change things up and begin burning off more fat:

- Cut out dairy products entirely, both low-fat and full fat

- Increase fat intake of healthy varieties

- Drop your carbohydrate daily intake even further

- Stop eating certain kinds of nuts and seeds (like cashews, which are highest in fat) or all kinds entirely

- Cut out gluten-containing products altogether, as well as gluten-contaminated (processes with gluten-containing foods even though it might not contain it itself) if you are sensitive to gluten

- Cut out sweeteners, including honey, syrups, and artificial sweeteners

- Track all your carbs and calories (macros in general) so you can make sure nothing is sneaking in

- Cut out processed foods

Progress isn't always about decreasing the number on the scale; for this reason, considering switching to measuring (chest, waist, thighs, upper arms) instead of weighing. This way you get a more accurate account of your progress.

Q: Should I take any supplement while on the Keto diet?

It's always a good idea to talk to a qualified medical professional on this subject, but because it's pretty common for people to get muscle cramps or just feel a bit off after starting a Ketogenic diet, there are some supplements that have been recommended to help with those issues. These supplements include:

- Multivitamins for your specific gender, condition, lifestyle, and age

- Mineral supplement that contains potassium, magnesium, and other trace minerals to support your electrolyte balance

- Vitamin B (full spectrum) Complex

- Vitamin D with Calcium Supplement

Consult your medical practitioner or nutritionist to address your individual needs.

Q: Is eating all this fat bad for me? What about heart attacks?

There are three known primary fat categories: saturated fats, polyunsaturated fats, and monounsaturated fats. In the past, we thought that saturated fats were responsible for a lot of rising health issues, and there seemed to be a lot that connected these fats to a plethora of health problems, specifically heart disease. In recent years, however, science has discovered that saturated fats are not to blame for heart attacks but can also help to improve cholesterol levels. Polyunsaturated fats, however, are a bit trickier to understand. Polyunsaturated fats are commonly found in processed foods and condiments, particularly those with hydrogenated vegetable oils, are notably unhealthy for a number of reasons, plus they usually have a lot of trans fats; trans fats have legitimately been connected to heart disease and other health issues (like obesity) and therefore should be avoided.

On the other hand, there are also polyunsaturated fats that occur naturally in certain foods, like fish and certain kinds of eggs, which are quite beneficial for us; these good fats have shown to help balance cholesterol levels, for example. So be sure to include sources of these healthy, naturally found kinds of fats, and try your best to eliminate the unnatural, unhealthy varieties. Lastly, we have monounsaturated fats. These are typically healthy and can be eaten without worry. Olive oil, for example, is more proportionately a monounsaturated fat, which is healthy for us and can help with lowering our cholesterol.

Q: Isn't fasting only a "fad" and can it really help me lose weight?

Fasting is not a fad as it has been utilized for thousands of years in medicine, various cultures and religions. It wasn't invented yesterday. In addition, fasting can help you lose weight and maintain it. The key is to find the fasting protocol that works best for you in conjunction with a low carbohydrate high-fat eating program to achieve the benefits you desire.

Q: Isn't fasting just another name for "starvation"?

While many may think so, fasting is not starvation. Fasting can be defined as a voluntary act of not eating for a specific time period.

Q: Won't you always be hungry with fasting? Will it cause you to overeat?

This is one of most asked questions as we have all experienced various weight loss programs where we are constantly hungry. First and foremost, if you eliminate processed foods and primarily eat whole foods (primarily transition to a low carbohydrate high-fat diet), the lowering of empty carbohydrates will help reduce your constant hunger pangs.

Because refined and highly processed foods have much of their fiber, essential nutrients, minerals and fats removed with sugar and other processed ingredients added back in, these types of carbohydrates enter quickly into your bloodstream where no satiety mechanisms are triggered to tell you that you are full. While this is occurring, your insulin levels skyrocket. When your insulin rises to a very high level, it indicates your body to store fat, but you are still hungry, so you eat more and store more fat. Thus, you are in a never-ending cycle of storing fat and continue to gain weight.

Such foods like fresh leafy green vegetables contain many nutrients and important fiber that triggers the satiety receptors as your stomach stretches. Both protein and fats trigger satiety mechanisms which also indicate when you are full to stop eating.

Q: I have never fasted before. Is it safe and is it hard to do?

As I previously mentioned, fasting has been around for thousands of years and one of the most used therapies in medicine. Fasting is not a new fad or something that appeared from nowhere. Therefore, it is safe if you first consult with your medical doctor and receive concurrence.

Believe it or not, you are fasting every night during your sleep. While it may be about 6 to 8 hours per night depending on your sleep patterns, your body is working to repair and rejuvenate itself for the next day.

Q: Don't you lose electrolytes with fasting?

There exist several discussions on loss of electrolytes and malnutrition during fasting, but the main issue is really about the deficiency of micronutrients. Studies have not found any evidence of malnutrition during prolonged fasts. Some of the key points are:

- Potassium levels only decreased slightly and without the use of any supplements

- Calcium, phosphorous and magnesium levels were stable as just about all the calcium and phosphorous are stored in our bones.

Q: Can you exercise when you are fasting?

Many believe that you should not exercise when fasting. There is no reason why you should not exercise unless you have some medical or physical condition preventing you. However, I suggest you start exercising once you transition to a fasting regimen for a couple of weeks, so your body becomes adapted to fasting. Start slow and progress with your exercise program over time. Don't be in a hurry. You are beginning a new healthy lifestyle change so don't overstress your body all at once. Exercise can be safely done with fasting but preferably during a fasted state for the best results.

Q: Can anyone fast?

Fasting can be done by many but there are exceptions. Children, the sick and elderly, underweight adults, pregnant and women breast-feeding, and those with serious medical conditions should not attempt fasting. Those who are on medications and have health issues must always speak to their doctor first before attempting to fast or start any new diet or physical exercise program.

Conclusion

Now that you have finished this book, it is only natural to be extremely anxious to get started not only with the Keto diet but with intermittent fasting as well. Nevertheless, it is important to follow the steps outlined in the chapters and start with the Keto diet before adding in intermittent fasting after your body has had the time it needs to adjust to the change, which should be a minimum of one month.

While you may be anxious to get started losing as much weight as possible, forcing your body to adapt to both lifestyle changes at once is likely to cause it to feel as though you are in a situation where it needs to hold on to every single calorie possible, curtailing weight loss in the process. Instead, it is important to give your body the time it needs to adjust and realize that following the Ketogenic diet while fasting intermittently is more akin to a marathon than a sprint which means that slow and steady wins the race.

Adhere to the outlined steps and make the journey a success. Good luck!

If you find this book helpful in anyway a review to support my endeavors is much appreciated.

Anti-Inflammatory Keto (30% More Effective)

Complete Beginners Guide to the Ketogenic Low-Carb Clarity with
Intermittent Fasting for Accelerated Results; Reset your Life Today and Slim
Down Forever

Christine Moore

CHRISTINE
MOORE

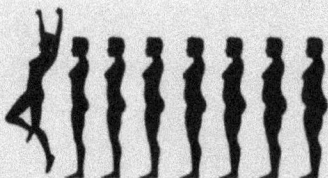

ANTI-INFLAMMATORY
KETO
30 PERCENT
MORE *Effective*

**COMPLETE WOMEN AND MEN BEGINNERS GUIDE TO THE
KETOGENIC LOW-CARB CLARITY WITH INTERMITTENT FASTING
FOR ACCELERATED WEIGHT LOSS: RESET YOUR LIFE TODAY**

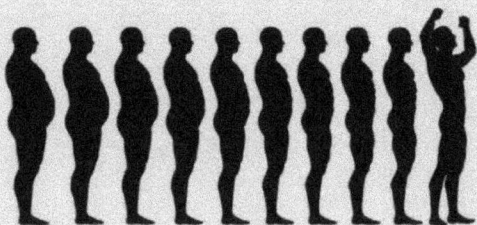

Introduction

If you are looking for a way to get healthier and eat better, then this is the right book for you. Health should always be one of our foremost concerns, with diet being one of the main factors that affect our health. Due to the booming food industry and consumerism, among other factors, our diets have undergone a very drastic and unhealthy change.

Our dietary choices are often influenced by advertisements and packaging that aim to financially benefit food corporations rather than human health. The widely available and extremely cheap junk food and processed food options found in supermarket shelves have directly contributed to unhealthy food choices and increased weight issues.

If you compare statistics from your grandparent's times to recent years, you will notice the increase in obesity, type 2 diabetes, eating disorders, among other health concerns. As a result of these issues, there is higher concern with healthy weight loss and dieting, but often people get caught up on fad diets that are not necessarily effective. The purpose of this book is to present information about the Keto-

Anti-Inflammatory Keto (30% More Effective)

Mediterranean diet and the many benefits associated with each diet individually, as well as the diets in combination with one another.

You may have heard of the Ketogenic and Mediterranean diets, even if you're not very familiar with the specifics of each. In this book, the details of each will be discussed, alongside, how they can improve your personal well-being and ways in which you can implement them.

These days' people have become more conscious of the ingredients that go in the preparation of their food. There is more awareness about all the harmful additives and preservatives in processed food. For this reason, the focus is shifting to eating more wholesome and natural food.

Through learning about the ketogenic diet, you will also learn how our ancestors ate and why following such a diet is still beneficial for our health today. Illness and weight issues were relatively non-existent in older times compared to now. Furthermore, the Mediterranean diet is a heart-friendly diet. These are not fad diets, and we have considered various factors before recommending them for the benefit of the reader. You don't have to stop eating everything you like or sit and count the ingredients in all you ate. You don't have to switch to a liquid diet or eat only once a day.

For many years, fat was considered the culprit behind increased weight concerns, but it is not true at all. Fat is an important part of your diet. So, stop listening to all the false information that you may be bombarded with. Instead, we will explain everything about the foods that will benefit your health and how you can switch to a healthy and still appealing diet.

It is very important to make conscious decisions about what you pick up at the store or and cook with. Good food choices will not only have a very significant impact on weight loss and management, but also improving overall physical and mental health. As you read on, you will learn how you can do this with the help of the Ketogenic Mediterranean diet. You will be able to eat good wholesome and delicious food that will benefit your health for years to come.

Chapter 1:
The Ketogenic Diet

This chapter will introduce the fundamentals of the Ketogenic (Keto) diet, how it works, and transitioning your body from running on carbohydrates (i.e. carbs) to running on fats. The ketogenic diet should be thought of more as a lifestyle; it doesn't set unrealistic and unhealthy rules about what you should or should not eat, or how much and how often. You won't have to curb your hunger with only boiled vegetables, or switch to raw shakes instead of wholesome meals.

The ketogenic lifestyle is not a demanding fad diet that will require immense self-control and stress you out about your food and weight. You won't have to starve yourself at any point either. This diet helps you understand what is good for your body and what is detrimental towards your health. You will automatically choose to make choices that will benefit you and not harm you.

The food corporations usually lie about the nutritious value about the foods they are trying to sell and make you believe that food labeled low fat or fat-free is healthy for you. All this is just a sham to mislead you and make you purchase their products. Recently, scientists and nutritionists have started endorsing the fact that our ancestors were much healthier than us and this was due to their healthier diets. The ketogenic diet recommends that we all shift back to that healthy diet again. There is a reason your grandma complains about what you constantly snack on. The older generations ate much more wholesome foods and thus managed to stay fit and healthy.

Our processed diets are doing nothing to benefit us. You must realize that everything you are told is not true, especially when it comes to the negative stigma that has become attached to fats. Most people in recent years have blamed fats as the main culprit behind any issues related to foods. But there are healthy fats that are essential for good health. Therefore, you should not follow any diets that eliminate fat from your food. Basing your food choices on correct facts or information is important.

If your main concern is excess weight, you need to understand the reason why you gained it in the first place. It is not always due to excessive eating but more about what you are eating. As mentioned already, it is not all due to fat either. The real culprit is the processed food that the food industry pushes for their profit and at the cost of our good health. The fat that occurs naturally in meat, dairy and other natural sources is good for health. The corporations are who have pushed the blame for bad health on fat for their benefit over the past couple of decades.

Anti-Inflammatory Keto (30% More Effective)

With the growing processed food industry, you will notice the rise in food-related issues as well. Type 2 Diabetes is one of the diseases that increased alarmingly with this. This was not the case even a few decades ago. You can see that fats are not the blame and instead you should eliminate unhealthy processed food from your diet. Another evil in your diet is sugar that must be removed or controlled. This ingredient causes only harm and has no nutritional benefit whatsoever for your health. Sugar and not fats can cause an alarming increase in your body weight too. You probably don't even realize how much-refined sugar is present in most of the processed food you consume. You can see how the industry has gained enough power to control our eating habits for their gain. When people notice that they gain weight, they start eating less or following fad diets. Instead of doing that, you can try to opt for healthier diet options like the ketogenic diet.

The ketogenic diet tells you to eat more like our ancestors, but with a decrease in the number of carbohydrates consumed while increasing the quantity of fats, thus pushing the body to burn fat as fuel. The purpose behind this strategy is to keep the body in a constant state of ketosis because, instead of banning fats from your diet, you will benefit more by majorly reducing your carbohydrate consumptions.

The demonization of fats is not going to help you in any way. Refined carbohydrates are more detrimental to your health and need to be reduced especially if you want to lose weight. Don't follow fad diets that leave you hungry for hours at a time. At some point, you will have to give in to hunger and then end up binge eating, fats help you feel full longer, preventing food cravings that can contribute to excess eating. You can eat all your regular meals with a heightened level of consciousness about the ingredients that you consume. The Keto also advocates for moderate consumption of proteins, which can also be obtained from wholesome and nutritious sources. There are many reports of people who have tried the keto diet found it to be helpful in losing weight, increasing stamina, and observing overall health improvements.

The ketogenic diet's name refers to the ketones and ketosis that occur in the human body as a result of the food that is consumed and used as the main source of energy. A constantly induced state of ketosis will help the body utilize stored fat for fuel; this includes excess fat stored in the liver, helping to reduce the likelihood of Fatty Liver Disease. The main thing that you learn from the ketogenic diet is that fats are not what cause obesity, heart attacks and all the other problems that they are usually blamed for. So, start adding them back into your diet liberally, if the fats that you decide to eat are from the right sources. You might be skeptical about this but take a chance, and you will not regret it.

Benefits of The Ketogenic Diet

Anti-Inflammatory Keto (30% More Effective)

Reducing carbohydrates will reduce excess triglycerides in the body. The keto diet helps in blood pressure regulation and will prevent heart issues and hardening of arteries as well.

High levels of insulin in the body can cause polycystic ovary syndrome in women. The ketogenic diet helps to reduce this excess insulin in the body and thus lowers risk of PCOD, which can be harmful to women and causes problems in conception and fertility.

You will also see that there is less occurrence of acid reflux or heartburn since these are increased by consumption of carbs like potatoes or foods containing sugars.

Certain studies show that the ketogenic diet benefits patients who have epilepsy and cancer; however, this is still being researched on, and no concrete evidence supports it.

Due to the benefits that the keto diet has on brain health, it can also reduce the risk of conditions like Alzheimer's or Parkinson's disease.

Another benefit is that the keto diet keeps a healthy check on uric acid levels in the body. If it is too much, it can cause gout or kidney stone formation, but the keto diet regulates it.

It is evident that there are a lot of benefits associated with following the ketogenic diet. For this reason, we recommend that you try the Keto diet for yourself.

Precautions

Before you follow any specific diet, you should consult a doctor. They will help you in deciding which diet is the most appropriate for your body and if there are any that might have a detrimental effect on your health. Every person's body is different and has its own needs. You cannot expect the same diet to work for every person and to have the same results. There are certain health issues or conditions as well that might make a certain diet or certain ingredients unsuitable for your body. Consultation from a doctor will help you to avoid any unwanted health issue aggravations. They will instead guide you so that you can reap the maximum benefit from the diet in a healthy way.

Note that those who have diseases related to the liver, kidney or pancreas should avoid the keto diet. The diet is also not suited for anyone who has muscular dystrophy. It is helpful for patients of diabetes type two and should not be followed by patients who have diabetes type one. Gestational diabetes does not react well with the ketogenic diet in the body.

Pregnant and nursing women have different nutritional requirements and should always consult their doctors as changing diets may affect their and their infant's health. Someone who suffers from eating disorders should always consult a doctor before following any specific diet. Their focus should be on regaining health, and the doctor will determine if the ketogenic diet is appropriate for such patients. Strict diets can often backfire for people with eating disorders when they should be focusing on healthier eating. These are just some precautions that we recommend you keep in mind before you start following the ketogenic diet or any such diet blindly. This diet is a safe and healthy diet that a lot of people have tried and benefited from; however, certain illnesses or conditions of the body require special care that you need to make sure you provide to stay healthy.

Side Effects of The Ketogenic Diet

As with any change in behavior, there may be some side effects when you initially start the keto diet. These side effects are usually temporary and pass over time and with care. Pay extra attention if you suffer from any medical conditions or take medications that might react adversely with the ketogenic diet.

One of the most common side effects is hypoglycemia, which causes dizziness, fatigue and irritability. This will pass after a few weeks, but to address it effectively, frequently eat small meals and stay hydrated throughout the day. Also, consider adding or maintaining enough sodium into your diet.

Other side effects can be caused by HPA axis dysfunction, which refers to the three glands; hypothalamus, pituitary and adrenal. You can deal with the associated condition with the help of apoptogenic herbs, blood sugar regulation and hydration.

Chapter 2:
Ketosis

In this chapter we talk about ketosis, how to achieve it, and the science behind it. To understand how the ketogenic diet works, you should have a basic understanding of the process of ketosis. You will get an overview of what ketosis is and how inducing it will benefit you.

Ketosis is the metabolic process of converting stored fat into energy. Normally, glucose is the primary source of energy, but during ketosis, stored fat is used instead. When fats are consumed, the body is prompted to burn them for fuel because more ketones are produced in the liver, and thus the body will use fats as its prime energy source. As the body continuously needs energy, it will constantly keep burning all the extra fat stored all around your body. When this is happening, you will soon see a difference in the shape of your body and a reduction in the number on the weighing scale.

Additionally, during constant ketosis, hunger is mostly satiated, and as such, you feel fuller for longer. With time, there are fewer cravings and hunger pangs, allowing you to feel satisfied between meals. Dealing with hunger pangs is a major issue with other diets that force you to eat less. It requires a lot of will power to follow those fad diets and ignore hunger pangs.

At some point or the other, most people end up binge eating after such diets. Binge eating usually involves carbohydrate-loaded food that will cause more weight gain; however, the ketogenic diet will curb this excess hunger healthily.

During ketosis, you will feel full for longer periods even while the body is burning off excess fat. It takes a little time to adapt to the diet initially, but over time you will be able to sustain it. Another benefit is that ketosis increases the level of good cholesterol in the body, which in turn decreases the level of bad cholesterol. The HDL levels tend to rise during ketosis, and it takes the LDL for processing in the liver. HDL is essential for certain functions in your body so don't assume that all cholesterol is bad. Focus more on reducing the carbohydrates that have a negative impact on your body. Many studies have been conducted over the years to see how the ketogenic diet and ketosis affect different people. People who frequently play sports experience increased stamina and have more energy to be active for a longer period. They usually turn to carb loading for energy, but energy for carbohydrates burns off very fast. Energy derived from fats takes longer to burn and thus provides energy for a longer time. The process of ketosis also showed improvement in focus and stamina of people. Although research is still being done to study the effects and benefits of the ketogenic diet, it is one of the best ways to lose weight and get healthier.

Let us understand ketosis and its benefit in a short and simple way. We are all aware that the body uses glucose as its main source of energy for the body. When you reduce the carbohydrates in the diet and increase the fats, there isn't enough carbohydrate to use for energy. The body now needs to adapt to survive this deficit of glucose, so it will start using the fats in the body for energy. When carbohydrates are in deficit, more ketones are produced in the liver. When these ketones are used up for energy, the stored fats are then burned for energy. Thus, you will see how the ketosis process helps you burn unwanted weight off your body and get back to a healthier size. Ketosis is a natural metabolic process that works automatically when you switch to the ketogenic diet. Ketosis induces the following benefits to the body:

Reduce Appetite
Ketosis reduces appetite by One of the worst effects of fad dieting is that it leaves you very hungry and unsatisfied. This will cause you to give up quite soon and end up eating more; however, ketosis will help you in reducing your appetite itself when your carbohydrate consumption also goes down.

Weight Loss

It will help you in losing weight quite fast compared to any other method of affecting the body to burn fat. During the first week after you start following the ketogenic diet, the body will lose water weight due to low carbohydrate consumption, which also decreases insulin levels. Afterwards, fat is burned off, which results in weight loss.

Burn Abdominal Fat

Ketosis helps to burn excess abdominal fat, which is usually one of the toughest areas for fat loss. Most people spend hours at the gym doing ab exercises to lose abdominal fat, but ketosis makes this much easier. The different places that fat is stored in your body will affect your health. This abdominal fat is usually associated with insulin resistance and inflammation and can cause metabolic dysfunction. Therefore, ketosis is very beneficial for your health in getting rid of this visceral fat that lodges around the organs.

Curb Triglycerides

Triglycerides are fat molecules that circulate in the blood. Ketosis reduces the level of triglycerides very significantly. People who lead more sedentary lifestyles will tend to have increased triglycerides, which increases the risk for heart disease. Consuming a diet with too little fats will increase the level of triglycerides while a low carb diet will reduce it.

Increased Lipoproteins

Ketosis will also aid in increasing levels of high-density lipoproteins in your body. This is the good kind of cholesterol that should be there in your body and should always be higher than the bad cholesterol or LDL.

Controlling Diabetes by Reducing Insulin and Blood Pressure
Ketosis reduces blood sugar and insulin in the body. As such, ketosis helps people who suffer from diabetes type two and insulin resistance. Furthermore, ketosis can help lower high blood pressure, which is a risk factor for different diseases related to the heart and kidney.

Ketosis is also beneficial for brain health since it burns ketones. Therefore, the ketogenic diet is used to induce ketosis in children with epilepsy who might not be responding to treatment by drugs.

As you can see, there are various reasons why the ketogenic diet is used to induce ketosis in the human body. This process can have many beneficial effects on health and easily help to lose excess weight, which is detrimental to the body. We will give you a straightforward breakdown on how to achieve ketosis, consider performing the following:

First, restrict your consumption of all forms of carbohydrates.

Then, limit your intake of proteins in order to lower the level of keto-sis. To lose weight, eat approximately 0.7 grams of protein per pound of your lean body mass.

You should stop worrying about and hating fat. In this diet, fats are your main source of fuel, and you should be consuming more of it without questioning yourself. Give it a chance; if you follow the guide-lines given in this book, you will be burning more fat than you con-sume.

You must remember to drink at least a gallon of water every day in order to maintain consistent hydration, ensuring regulation of vital bodily functions and controlling hunger.

Avoid snacking in order to decrease insulin spikes throughout the day, allowing for quicker weight loss. Eating too often will slow down the process of weight loss.

Practice intermittent fasting, which fasting. In another chapter of this book, you will learn about intermittent fasting and its benefits. Fasting has been known to increase the levels of ketones in the blood.

Exercise daily for at least 30 to 40 minutes. You might start with walking to build up your stamina, aiming to achieve high-intensity workouts with time. Exercising helps to regulate blood sugar levels and aids in weight loss. Even if you reach your goal weight, continue to exercise to maintain a healthy weight and activity level.

Check the ingredients on the labels of any food you purchase in order to avoid unwanted carbohydrates, additives, and preservatives that are bad for your health.

Now that you've learned how to induce ketosis, keep an eye out for the following symptoms that indicate you are maintaining ketosis:

- You will notice increased urination compared to before. Keto acts like a natural diuretic that will increase the frequency of urination in your body. The acetoacetate ketone body will also be excreted in urine, and this can cause the frequency of urination.

- You might notice that your mouth has turned dry and you will feel constantly thirsty. The increased urination dehydrates the body and requires that you keep drinking enough water to replenish the electrolytes required by the body.

- One side effect of ketosis is what is known as keto breath, which results from the metabolism of acetone, a type of ketone. Acetone is found in nail polish remover, and you may find your breath smells like that for a while. Energy levels will increase while your appetite will decrease because fats take longer to metabolize, and as such, keep you energized for a longer period.

These are just some of the common symptoms that you will be able to notice over time as you continue the ketogenic diet. They will indicate that the process of ketosis is working. You do not have to stress yourself out with a lot of testing and measuring to check if you are losing weight. Trust the process and keep track of your progress to understand if you are doing something wrong. Place your focus on the nutritional part of your diet and eat the right kinds of foods within limits set by the diet in terms of macros. There is no calorie counting or portion restriction, so it is simple for anyone to follow.

Chapter 3:
The Nutritional Break Down

The following chapter will include the nutritional break down of the Keto diet, and elaborate on the percentages of fats, protein and carbohydrates that should be consumed.

The ketogenic diet reduces carbohydrate intake to the minimum amount required for good health, thus eliminating any additional adverse carbohydrates from your diet. It also increases fat consumption significantly and promotes moderate consumption of proteins, improving muscle health. The diet is more flexible than one might realize, ensuring that every individual gets the nutrition his or her body needs.

There are several variations of the ketogenic diet that can be chosen according to everyone's needs.

Standard Ketogenic Diet

Standard ketogenic diet (SKD) allows very little carbohydrate consumption with moderate amounts of protein and a high quantity of fats. The typical breakdown is 75% fats, 20% proteins and 5% carbohydrates.

High Protein Keto

High protein ketogenic diet is, as the name indicates, includes an increased amount of proteins. The typical breakdown of this version is 60% fats, 35% proteins, and 5% carbohydrates.

Cyclical Ketogenic Diet

Cyclical ketogenic diet (CKD) allows for higher amounts of carbohydrates for a few days, followed by days of strict ketogenic diet. Typically, it includes two days of high carbohydrate intake, followed by five days of keto diet in the week.

Targeted Ketogenic Diet

Targeted ketogenic diet (TKD) is designed for people who have high levels of activity, allowing for increased carbohydrates near workout times.

If you consider the template calorie-wise, the ketogenic diet will provide 60-75% of your required calories from fats, about 15-30% of calories are sourced from proteins and carbohydrates only provide 5-10% of calories.

Usually, people who want to lose weight follow the standard ketogenic version or the high protein ketogenic diet. The other two versions are focused on accommodating the needs of athletes or as more advanced versions. The standard ketogenic version is the most highly recommended version for the user to follow. Usually, the Keto diet allows 20 to 30 grams of net carbs, but this limit can be adjusted with time. For those seeking to lose weight, it is important to keep track of the total and net carbs consumed. Net carbohydrates are the carbohydrates in food that can be digested and used for energy. Since the human body cannot digest fiber or sugar alcohols, these are not included in the calculation. The total carbohydrate count, on the other hand, includes all carbohydrates consumed. The recommended net carbohydrate limit is no more than 25 grams per day, and the total carbohydrate limit is 35 grams per day.

Proteins should be consumed according to the overall calorie requirement, and the rest of the diet should be filled with healthy fats. For instance, if your total calorie intake per day is around 1800 calories, then you must ensure that about 1300-1400 calories are in the form of fats, about 250-300 calories from proteins and the rest from carbs.

The ketogenic diet is focused on controlling the macronutrients, also known as macros, in your diet. Macros are a part of every person's diet, and they include the fats, proteins and carbohydrates. You already know the restriction placed on carbohydrate consumption and the specification for how much proteins and fats you should consume on this diet.

The exact numbers of calories can be determined by checking various factors, such as age, gender, daily activity level, body fat percentage, height, and weight. There should also be a goal, a quantifiable desired outcome that will increase motivation throughout the process. All these factors together will determine the quantity of each required macro and the other nutrients that need to be provided to their body as a part of their daily diet.

Chapter 4:
Dirty Keto

Dirty keto is a recently popularized version of the keto diet that follows the same macronutrient breakdown but is not concerned with the sources of the macronutrients. As a result, vital micronutrients that essential for good health are missing in the dirty keto diet.

The dirty keto diet does assist in weight loss, but results in unpleasant side effects, such as bloating, inflammation and hunger pangs. Once the diet is concluded, the weight returns. The dirty keto version is suitable for certain situations, such as travel, or adjusting as needed. But ultimately, the ketogenic diet with home cooking is the best healthy method to follow. If you are worried about sacrificing the variety of foods you eat outside, you will be surprised by how many keto recipes there are for you to try out. They are much healthier and will help you lose weight in the long term.

The dirty keto version of the ketogenic diet is another version you can consider. Lately, it has gained a lot of popularity because it claims to help you lose weight even while you eat junk food. Who doesn't dream of eating junk food and still staying fit? Therefore, a lot of people are trying this version of the ketogenic diet out; it is appealing to many. But there are a lot of things to consider dirty keto. Here we will weigh the pros and cons and see if you really should try this version of the diet.

The ketogenic diet minimizes carbohydrate intake and increases fat so that the body uses fats as its source of fuel. The ketogenic diet might not be a sustainable, long-term diet, although it is very beneficial for losing weight.

The dirty keto diet allows for binge eating junk food for meals if the carbohydrate content is kept at a minimum. As a result, you may not be obtaining the necessary nutrients, healthy fats and macronutrients your body requires. People may end up eating a lot of butter, bacon, cheese and other foods that are technically keto-friendly as they are high in fats; but they are also high in cholesterol and can have a negative impact on your health. Excessive consumptions of such food can significantly increase the risk of heart diseases.

Some versions of dirty keto meals include steaks smothered with butter, mounds of cheddar cheese on enchiladas that are low in carbs, etc. You might lose weight when you switch to this dirty keto version, but it is an unhealthy choice. You will be consuming only unhealthy food as your meal replacements, and these will have no health benefits other than losing weight. The term "dirty keto" is just another way to refer to the fast and dirty way of eating packaged and processed foods instead of wholesome home-cooked meals. The only advantage of the dirty keto diet is that it is convenient.

The ketogenic diet already removes carbohydrates in a major way from your diet. When you switch to dirty keto, you will also be removing all the healthy foods that will sustain your body and keep it in good form for a long time. Sole focus on macronutrients from the dirty keto diet will result in a deficiency of nutrients that are nourishing for your gut. Your digestive system requires certain resistant starches, prebiotic fibers, etc. that are only supplied when you eat a healthy planned diet that contains the required components like vegetables. These are essential for good gut health, and if you neglect them, you will surely see the detrimental effects it has on your health. The keto diet ensures a holistic approach to food that ensures all the nutrients your body needs are met, while the dirty keto diet usually results in deficiencies due to the lack of focus and thoughtful consideration of meals. The dirty keto diet often contains foods high in saturated fats, which are pro-inflammatory and linked to hearts diseases and diabetes. The usual ketogenic diet will encourage you to eat vegetables and starchy food that is healthy for you; however, all these components are removed in the dirty keto version. It won't benefit you to substitute buns for some lettuce in your burger. You are still only eating junk food that does not provide nutrients to your diet. The clean keto diet will help you cook with healthy fats like coconut oil, olive oil or butter but in the dirty keto diet, you will be wallowing in pork rinds.

Despite such factors, a lot of people would prefer to try the dirty keto diet to lose weight. The dirty keto diet tends to be more appealing because it can be very difficult to make permanent and real changes in diet and lifestyle, requiring effort and self-education. It has much easier rules to follow, and allows for junk food, and as a result, it only achieves short-term gains at the best, with no move towards a long-term healthy body and lifestyle. This is where you must decide if you want the long-term benefits of the standard ketogenic diet or the short-term weight loss benefits of the dirty keto diet.

The regular or clean keto diet will provide you with 5% calories from carbs, 75-90% calories from fats and 6-25% calories from fats. The numbers can be adjusted within these given ranges. But the dirty keto diet does not include any specifications to determine and ensure you have obtained the required macronutrients and there are no guidelines for healthy food suggestions. You can go to any fast food restaurant and simply opt out of the carbohydrate ingredients. Dirty keto can be a very tempting alternative for those who love fast food or hate to cook. It can be an option when you occasionally eat out to choose such dirty keto friendly options; however, if you eat junk food for all your meals, your system will suffer. However, the quality of the food you eat is more important than eating for the sake of eating or losing weight; the quality of food directly impacts your health. Therefore, the dirty keto version is not what anyone would recommend for long-term use. You need to think carefully about your diet and make sure it contains all the required sources of fiber, minerals, vitamins, etc.

When you try the ketogenic diet, you should opt for the version that is clean, holistic and recommends healthy foods while removing processed, unhealthy products.

Dairy and Meats in Keto

A lot of people wonder if they should eat dairy products or meat during a ketogenic diet. Some dairy foods and meat are keto friendly while others are not and should be reduced or eliminated. The food and quantity will be determined by your body, goals, and factors such as lactose intolerance.

With regards to dairy foods, products like condensed milk or yogurts that have sugar added are not keto-friendly. Instead, you could eat ghee, butter, and hard cheeses. Certain foods that have a lot of fats are ideal for keto diet. Ghee and butter can be used for cooking since they are nearly exclusively composed of fat. For those who are lactose intolerant, ghee is a suitable alternative to butter. If your aim is to lose weight, you will simply have to monitor how much ghee or butter you consume.

In considering cheeses, certain types are much lower in carbohydrates and are thus keto-friendly. However, the exact type of cheese should be considered in order to determine the specific macros, and thus overall benefit. Typically, parmesan, gouda, brie, goat cheese, mozzarella, feta, and cheddar varieties are quite low in carbohydrates. Avoid specialty cheeses that have added ingredients such as fruit, which are quite high in carbohydrates. Generally, if you don't over-indulge on cheese, it is usually a keto-friendly ingredient.

As an ingredient, milk can be substituted with heavy cream (the better option) or half and half in desserts or coffees. These dairy products are more keto-friendly than milk since they contain a relatively low amount of carbohydrates. Try to use real heavy cream, which is about 40% fat and unsweetened. However, if you have a serious dairy intolerance, cut them out of your diet.

In dairy products, fat can range from no fat (0%) to total fat (100%). Fat can be saturated or unsaturated; note that some foods can contain both, forming a complex form of natural fat, which can benefit your health. Dairy products also contain many micronutrients like vitamin D, vitamin B12, and calcium, which are required by the body.

When you are trying to lose weight, it might help to cut down on dairy products and tracking your consumption since they are very easy to overeat and as a result, cause significant weight gain if consumed in excess. If you are facing difficulty in adapting to fat as your body's main source of fuel, or you've reached a plateau in weight loss, you might consider going dairy-free for a while. You should also consider it if you want to balance some autoimmune condition or have digestive issues such as diarrhea.

Ultimately, most dairy products are keto-friendly, so you can continue eating them in healthy versions of food. Don't overload on cheese if you are on a dirty keto diet since it will just make you gain more weight.

Now let's talk about meat. Usually, most diets will instruct you to opt for leaner meats such as chicken breast, and you are expected to give up fatty steaks and pork. The keto diet does not impose this restriction, but rather encourages greasy meats in moderation. Meat contains a lot of protein, which can take you out of the state of ketosis that the ketogenic diet aims to induce. Therefore, you cannot have a very meat heavy keto diet. They are okay to consume in moderation, but they should not be a staple in your everyday meals.

The leaner cuts of meat that other diets recommend include chicken breasts, but these are very high in protein. If you want to achieve ketosis, you cannot eat too much proteins. The main reason is that the body converts protein into glucose through a process called gluconeogenesis, which means that eating high amounts of protein will increase your body's glucose levels. This would be counterproductive to the ketogenic diet and will prevent ketosis. Your body will use the protein for glucose and then the glucose for energy. The fats will stay stored and will add to your weight. Therefore, on the keto diet, only one-fifth of your meal should consist of protein. Therefore, incorporate mostly non-meat sources of fat in your meals in order to avoid gluconeogenesis. This does not mean you cannot eat meats; however, do so sparingly. In terms of good fat to protein ratio, the meats that are allowed include fatty steaks, such as ribeye and brisket, unprocessed and nitrate-free bacon, chicken thighs with skin, fatty fish like salmon, and organ meats like liver or heart. Be sure to consider the protein content and omit them from your regular diet. Instead opt for animal fats such as lard or bacon grease, ghee, and eggs.

Chapter 5:
The Mediterranean Diet

In this chapter, we will discuss what the Mediterranean diet is and how it will benefit your health.

The Mediterranean diet is a very heart-healthy diet plan that is based on recipes from Mediterranean cuisine. It comprises of foods that people from countries around the Mediterranean, such as Italy, Greece eat. Research has shown that their diets were exceptionally healthy with minimal reported diseases that are prevalent these days and are related specifically to food and lifestyle. The studies also show that the Mediterranean diet aids in weight loss, and can reduce the risk of heart diseases, Type 2 diabetes, and even premature death.

The diet incorporates basic healthy eating practices alongside olive oil or red wine added to the meal. These are just some of the components that characterize Mediterranean cooking and make it flavor-full yet healthy. Although all healthy diets recommend nearly the same wholesome fruit, vegetables, whole grains, certain subtle variations make a difference. This variation seems to contribute to decreased levels of LDL and reduces the risk of heart diseases, cancer, Alzheimer's and Parkinson's diseases, and breast cancer. This diet helps to lower the level of LDL or bad cholesterol that is likely to build up in your arteries and cause issues. The Mediterranean diet is also not limited to one type of food or one form of cuisine. It encompasses many countries that surround the Mediterranean Sea, and thus you get to try a wide variety of dishes to select from. The Mediterranean diet is characterized by a high intake of plant-based foods, olive oil, moderate consumption of fish or poultry, and relatively low intake of dairy, red meats, sweets, and processed foods. Red wine is consumed in moderation as an accompaniment to a meal and is considered beneficial to the heart. There is a strong focus on communal meals in which everyone eats together, emphasizing the social and cultural aspects of the society. They also tend to rest after meals and are quite active on a regular basis. Due to westernization, however, there has been an increase in processed food within the Mediterranean countries, contributing to increased health concerns.

In the Mediterranean lifestyle, daily physical activity also plays an important role. It helps to maintain and attain the overall good health of every individual. You can try some regular running or aerobics or other activities that are more leisurely such as walking or just taking the stairs. Another easy way to stay active is to do some physical work around the house like cleaning or yard work. Anything that keeps you moving and active will benefit your health and especially your heart health. It will also aid in losing weight over time.

The Mediterranean diet is not just another hype diet and has scientific evidence to prove that it is beneficial for health. It is known to lower mortality, morbidity, cancer risk, cardiovascular disease, obesity, cognitive disease, metabolic syndrome, etc. Studies also show that patterns of the Mediterranean diet can help in the prevention or control of non-communicable diseases that are related to diet. The better the knowledge and access to healthy food, the higher the chances of the person staying disease free. According to the Mediterranean diet, you should emphasize the following:

- Eat more plant-based foods like vegetables, fruit, whole grains, nuts and legumes

- Use canola oil or olive oil instead of butter

- Eat fish or poultry about two times a week

- Use herbs and spices instead of salt to flavor food

- Eat red meat no more than two times a month

- Eat meals with family and friends

- Accompany your meal with a glass of red wine

- Exercise regularly

- Don't eat processed foods, added sugars, or refined grains

- Avoid trans fats from margarine or other processed foods

- Avoid low fat, diet and processed foods

Foods Found in the Mediterranean Diet

Traditionally, the Mediterranean diet includes a lot of fruit, rice, vegetables and pasta with fewer animal-sourced foods. The Mediterranean diet includes:

- Vegetables: tomatoes, broccoli, spinach, onions, cauliflower, cucumbers, kale, etc.

- Fruit: apples, bananas, melons, peaches, figs, dates, grapes, etc.

- Nuts: almonds, hazelnuts, walnuts, etc.

- Seeds: pumpkin seeds, sunflower seeds, etc.

- Legumes: beans, pulses (i.e. dried seeds of legumes), peanuts, peas, etc.

- Tubers: turnips, sweet potatoes, potatoes, etc.

- Eggs: chicken, duck or quail.

- Whole grains: brown rice, rye, corn, buckwheat, whole oats, etc.

- Fish or seafood: crab, trout, salmon, shrimp, oysters, etc.

- Poultry: duck, turkey or chicken.

- Dairy: cheese, Greek yogurt, etc.

- Herbs and spices: nutmeg, mint, rosemary, pepper and cinnamon.

- Healthy fats from avocados, olives, olive oil, etc.

- Water to stay hydrated.

- Tea and coffee (as you want without added sugars) and avoiding processed juices and beverages.

Benefits of The Mediterranean Diet

The Mediterranean diet is a healthy and nutritious diet that improves your quality of life and wellbeing without placing any extreme limits on your diet and allowing you to continue enjoying delicious foods. As you adapt to Mediterranean dietary habits, you will soon notice the benefits it has on your heart, brain, and overall health and longevity. Following are elaborations on some of the benefits of the Mediterranean diet on your body and mind:

Reduces the Risk of Type 2 Diabetes.

Many studies have demonstrated that the Mediterranean diet is highly beneficial for those who with diabetes or high blood pressure because it emphasizes foods with more monounsaturated fats and fiber. As a result, blood sugar levels and cholesterol decrease, aiding in the management of Type 2 diabetes. Replacing saturated or trans fats with unsaturated fats also assist in regulating insulin sensitivity.

Improves Heart Health

The incidence of heart diseases is low in Mediterranean countries compared to the United States, mainly due to the difference in dietary choices and activity level. They also drink a glass of red wine daily, and this also benefits heart health.

Maintains Agility with Age

Since this diet provides your body with all the nutrients it requires, alongside physical activity, there is a reduction in the risk of muscle weakness and frailty that occur with age. This diet has shown to reduce this risk of weakening muscles by more than half in people above 60. +

Reduces the Risk of Parkinson's Disease

The Mediterranean diet incorporates high amounts of antioxidants, which can reduce the risk of Parkinson's disease. These antioxidants are obtained from the fresh fruits and vegetables, seafood and healthy fat sources. Furthermore, antioxidants protect cells from oxidative stress, which can cause damage and promote the development of Parkinson's disease. Oxidation is a very common process that takes place in the body. On the other hand, oxidative stress occurs due to an imbalance between antioxidants and free radicals present in the body. When the body is functioning optimally, then these free radicals help fight off pathogens. When the number of free radical's present exceeds the number of antioxidants present, then the free radicals start to damage the DNA, proteins and other fatty tissues within the body. All this can lead to several illnesses over time if left unchecked.

Reduces the Risk of Alzheimer's Disease

As a result of the diet contributing to decreased cholesterol and blood sugar levels, the overall health of blood vessels improves, therefore reducing the risk of Alzheimer's, dementia, and other cognitive impairments. In this way, the quality of life can be preserved due to limited occurrences of burdensome illnesses.

Encourages Healthy Weight Loss

One primary advantage of the Mediterranean diet is that it is very easy to maintain long-term since it is not unreasonably restrictive and allows you to eat enough to satisfy your hunger, and thus stay satiated longer. The addition of regular exercise will allow you to lose weight steadily over time in a way that can be managed more easily for a longer period of time, which is a part of the Mediterranean lifestyle, and so you will see major weight loss if you stick to the diet for a longer time. Diets that allow you to lose weight too quickly are usually unhealthy and not sustainable. The Mediterranean diet encourages the body to slowly but steadily lose unhealthy weight in a way that can be managed for the long term.

Helps Fight Cancer

Research has shown that the Mediterranean diet can reduce the risk of cancer from developing, as well as cancer-related mortality. There seems to be some probable protective role against cancer that is played by the Mediterranean diet. More specifically, this diet is considered helpful in the prevention of the occurrence of breast cancer in women post menopause. This is especially beneficial since this breast cancer usually has a poor prognosis.

Maintains Cognitive Health

It is considered that following the Mediterranean diet will reduce the risk of development of degenerative diseases like Parkinson's or dementia. Studies have indicated that following this diet can improve a person's cognitive abilities by enhancing memory and improving focus and attention. This diet is also considered beneficial for progressing the language capabilities of the brain, which can assist in preventing dementia as well as maintaining general healthy brain function. This will help in better performance at work, better mental health and overall improvement in the quality of life.

Encourages Relaxation

The Mediterranean diet is not just a meal plan but a lifestyle. The meals are a very social experience, with a lot of time spent outside or exercising in one way or another. This lifestyle improves stress management and relaxation, allowing them to sleep better, have more energy and form better relationships.

Improves Mood Swings

Hectic and unhealthy lifestyles often cause mental health issues like depression, anxiety and mood swings. The Mediterranean diet has shown to have brain-boosting effects that help alleviate such symptoms and improve mental health. When the brain doesn't have enough dopamine hormone, these disorders tend to occur since this hormone is responsible for mood regulation, thought processing and body movements. The healthy foods encouraged by this diet ensure enough production of this chemical so that your mood remains elevated and happy. It also contributes to good gut health, which is also linked to mood triggers. Mental health disorders require proper treatment, but the diet acts as an effective aid for prevention as well as control.

Helps Fight Inflammation

The Mediterranean diet has been shown to reduce and regulate inflammation in the body, as well as any conditions that might arise from chronic inflammation. Oxidative stress is a major trigger for inflammation, but it can be reduced with antioxidants. If you eat more of foods containing choline, then you can further increase this positive impact Consuming more egg yolks, soybean, beets, and spinach will help to reduce inflammation.

Improves Skin

Your skin is highly impacted by your diet, so many doctors will recommend diet changes for people suffering from various skin conditions. The olive oil used in Mediterranean cooking contains a lot of vitamin E and antioxidants, which help to hydrate and nourish the skin. Red wine also contains resveratrol, which inhibits the growth of acne-causing bacteria. Another staple in the Mediterranean diet is tomato, which protects skin cells from cancer caused by exposure to the sun's ultraviolet rays.

Helps Relieve Pain

Since the Mediterranean diet consists of foods such as whole grains that are rich in magnesium, as well as fruit and vegetables that are rich in fiber, it naturally provides a means to assist in pain management, especially for those who suffer from chronic pain. This diet reduces inflammation, which can make a big difference in managing and reducing, and as such, alleviating stress. To benefit more from this pain-relieving aspect, you should increase your intake of foods that are rich in magnesium as it is proven to fight muscle pain. So, try to eat more of nuts, seeds, leafy greens, lentils, whole grains and beans.

Benefit Fertility

Studies showed that women who followed the Mediterranean diet were more fertile than women who followed a normal balanced diet and even demonstrated higher fertility after they switched to this diet. This diet can also benefit men in developing healthier sperm to increase likelihood of conception.

Increases Longevity

Between 1960 and 1990, mortality statistics showed that the people who lived in the Mediterranean region lived longer and the major contributing factor for this was their diet. The Mediterranean lifestyle can help you live longer, healthier and happier when all the aspects of their daily life are adapted.

Chapter 6:
Ketogenic Mediterranean Diet

In this chapter, you will learn how to combine the ketogenic diet with the Mediterranean diet. Both the diet's benefits that can easily assist any individual in losing weight and improving overall health by developing a more nutritious diet and active lifestyle.

The Mediterranean diet is a very widely accepted nutritional regime due to its evident health benefits from the macronutrient composition of the food and the active lifestyle. These contribute significantly to the health of the people who consume the Mediterranean diet, and thus they benefit from the most health benefits possible.

When it comes to losing weight, the ketogenic diet is a viable option to achieve any set weight goals. The ketogenic diet has a strong basis both physiologically and biochemically, allowing it to be useful for weight loss and heart health. Merging the ketogenic diet with the Mediterranean diet can have some of the best possible outcomes for someone who practices it appropriately.

Solely following the ketogenic diet often results in an imbalanced intake of fats due to the increased consumption of trans fats, saturated fats, or omega6 acids., and not enough intake of monosaturated fats and omega-3 fatty acids that are good for heart health.

By itself, the ketogenic diet inadvertently causes a heightened focus on macronutrients and too little focus on the micronutrients. When the food quality and micronutrient density is not enough or appropriate, you may face issues like hormone dysregulation, inflammation, and weight stalls. It also does not incorporate foods such as non-starchy vegetables, fatty fish, and virgin olive oil, which are included in the Mediterranean diet. The nutrient density, and active lifestyle of the Mediterranean diet can be combined with the standard ketogenic diet to lose weight and maximize health benefits.

Merging the two diets together will consist of olive oil, green vegetables, avocados, coconut oil, fish, eggs, cheese and lean meat, and a moderate consumption of red wine. Whole grains, starchy vegetables like potatoes, corn or peas, legumes and any food containing sugar or flour are eliminated.

The Keto-Mediterranean diet does not include fruit, even though it is a healthy food choice, due to the sugar fruits contain. The main emphasis is on using olive oil, fish, healthier fat and red wine. These are the few essential components that are common to the diet of all the people around the Mediterranean region. This is what differentiates this diet from other forms of the keto diet. A lot of evidence has demonstrated that combining the two diets can be very effective in reducing unhealthy appetites and unwanted weight, as well as being beneficial for people who suffer from heart disease, diabetes, and epilepsy. The Keto-Mediterranean diet can also help to reduce fasting glucose levels, prevent insulin resistance, cholesterol and triglycerides.

Olive oil is the main component of the Mediterranean diet that should be included in your diet due to its health benefits. Olive oil reduces the risk associated with most cardiovascular disease by influencing factors such as lipoprotein profile, glucose metabolism and blood pressure. It also reduces inflammation, oxidative stress and endothelial function. These positive effects are usually attributed to the monounsaturated fatty acids found within oil olive, especially extra virgin olive oil. Compounds like hydrocarbons, sterols, and polyphenols have demonstrated antioxidant, anti-inflammatory and even hypolipidemic properties. Studies have shown that a diet that is rich in monounsaturated fats will prevent both central fat redistribution and insulin resistance that is usually induced when the diet is rich in carbohydrates.

Red wine consists of phenolic compounds (this lends certain foods their red color) and ethanol, and these phenolic compounds are what contribute to the associated protection against cardiovascular diseases. Consuming red wine is beneficial due to the antiatherogenic properties of the antioxidant polyphenols. This combination also has a positive effect on hemodynamics. The amount of wine that should be consumed, if at all, varies with everyone, who should consult with his or her doctor first.

Fish contain three active components: docosahexaenoic acid, eicosatetraenoic acid, and two long chain omega-3 PUFA. Studies have shown that people who consume a lot of fish in their diets have lower rates of coronary heart disease. However, the consumption of fish should be limited as they may contain high levels of mercury, which is harmful to human health. Large fish with longer lifespans, like sharks or swordfish, have higher concentrations of omega-3 in their tissues, whereas smaller fish lower concentrations. The high concentration of omega 3 in fish helps increase insulin sensitivity and reduce inflammation. Saturated fats have a higher tendency to get stored as fat in the body while mono or polyunsaturated fats are more effectively used in fat oxidation.

Generally, people have the misconception that eating more fats and protein in their diet will cause excessive weight gain; however, studies conducted with the ketogenic Mediterranean diet proved that this diet is very effective in reducing weight and dealing with obesity. Unlike most other diets, the Keto-Mediterranean diet does not impose any calorie restrictions, although it does recommend avoiding overeating. The reason behind this effectiveness of the ketogenic Mediterranean diet is the synergy between the high protein keto nature and the MUFA (Monounsaturated fats) as well as PUFA (Polyunsaturated fats) in the Mediterranean diet. A lot of studies have confirmed that compared to other conventional low carbohydrate diets, the ketogenic diet is much more effective in treating obesity. A diet with high-unsaturated fat is also quite effective in preserving lean mass compared to a diet that is low in fats or carbohydrates. Studies also demonstrated that the ketogenic Mediterranean diet improves fasting glycemic index quite significantly. Since the diet also significantly reduced total cholesterol, LDL cholesterol, triacylglycerol's, etc. it creates a very positive cardiovascular profile. Red wine plays an important role in this last point as it also helps to increase levels of good cholesterol or HDL. Ultimately, you can see that all the factors of the ketogenic as well as the Mediterranean diet play an important role in the overall improvement of health and not just in losing weight. It is important to remember that the Mediterranean lifestyle plays a crucial role and not the just the food so imbibing it into your daily life would also be important if you were to follow the ketogenic Mediterranean diet.

As you read on, you will learn more about what foods you should or should not eat in the Ketogenic Mediterranean diet. The following are some tips to help you in the process of switching to this diet.

Reduce or eliminate the "white" foods, such as bread, pasta, cereals, rice and potatoes, because they all refined foods filled with starchy carbohydrates. Instead, switch to beans, lentil, and quinoa since these are healthy and quite filling as well. Also, limit the consumption of brown rice although it does not have to be eliminated.

Completely eliminate any sugar, sweetened drinks, and other sweetened foods because it is not beneficial to your health and mainly has adverse effects, such as weight gain, obesity and diabetes. There are a lot of keto-friendly desserts that you can opt for instead.

Consume as many vegetables as you can, adding a variety of colors on your plate, especially dark, leafy greens. Eat non-starchy vegetables as they will help increase your vital phytonutrient consumption. Phytonutrients are certain compounds that are essential to keep your body working properly and there are more than 25,000 types of phytonutrients present in plant-based foods. However, the most important of all are carotenoids, ellagic acid, flavonoids, resveratrol, phytoestrogens and glycosylates. By consuming keto-friendly plant-based produce, your body will be able to obtain all these necessary phytonutrients. There are a variety of recipes that you can try to make your meals healthy and delicious at the same time while using these ingredients.

Regularly add at least one to two ounces of a high-quality protein sources in your diet because your body requires a constant intake of protein since it is not stored internally. This will help you prevent muscle loss and reduce unhealthy appetites. Limit your consumption of processed meats. High-quality sources of protein include seafood, soy, oily fish, meat, tofu, chickpeas, lentils, nuts, and quinoa.

Eat one portion of fruit per day instead of processed or unhealthy snacks. You may select options like berries and pears. You should eat the fruits with edible peels since that is where most of the nutrients lie. Reduce intake of tropical fruits that are high in sugar, such as mangoes and bananas.

Don't cut out full-fat dairy products from your diet. There is a misguided fear that they are not good for your health or weight, but in fact, it is the opposite. You may even eat dairy such as cheese that might be high in calories, since it will keep you full for longer and provide fuel for energy.

Consume healthy fats and oils, like olive oil, in order to improve the absorption of essential fat-soluble vitamins.

Add vinegar to your diet because it can help in the process of weight loss, burning off abdominal fat, improving insulin sensitivity, and reducing blood sugar spikes after meals.

Stay hydrated by drinking plenty of water. There is no fixed quantity of water that everyone must drink, and while some should drink more, others might require less water for good health. Keep your body size, metabolic rate and rate of daily activity in mind as you determine your appropriate water content.

Save desserts for special occasions, and don't overindulge.

Control your portion size during meals so that you don't overeat. You could eat five small meals in a day rather than three larger meals; this is helpful because frequent meals can help curb unhealthy cravings. You can still stick to the breakfast-lunch-dinner routine but eat just enough to satiate your appetite. If you are hungry between meals, eat small portions of some keto-friendly snacks.

Studies show that people who strictly follow the Ketogenic Mediterranean diet have a significantly lower body mass index. It is an effective alternative to low-fat diets that are usually followed but don't work. This diet also has a much better effect on glycemic control and the lipids in the body.

Although there is no limit on calorie intake, moderation is key if you want to lose excess weight. Eating excessively will always cause weight gain regardless of the diet you follow and will strain your digestive system. This does not mean you can't have a slice of birthday cake at a party, but you should limit the size and minimize intake. You can always have a glass of wine or a pint of beer with your friends but limit it to no more than two. As we said, moderation will play an important role while you still enjoy a delicious and healthy diet.

If you are following the Ketogenic Mediterranean diet to lose or maintain weight, visit a doctor or professional to determine what your healthy weight range is. This range is determined based on your height, age, and overall health, and should be your guide. If your current weight is above the recommended healthy weight range, then you may have to put extra effort in cutting back on extra food, as well as adding more exercise into your daily routine.

Since the Keto-Mediterranean diet does not require counting calories, you shouldn't experience pressure, and hopefully will be more likely to succeed. Thankfully, this diet does not require any such thing, and thus you will feel less likely to fail. Just follow the guidelines given in this book and practice moderation. This will help you to lose your excess weight and stay healthy in the long term. In the case of pregnant women or children, we recommend consultation from a doctor to determine what the exact dietary requirements are for optimum health.

Chapter 7:
Keto-Mediterranean Vegetables

The Keto-Mediterranean diet features a variety of ingredients from all around the Mediterranean Sea that can be easily adaptable to your daily meals.

Vegetables should be eaten with every meal since they are very important sources of vitamins, fiber, nutrients, minerals and antioxidants. They are also great snacks to maintain satiety between meals and can be drizzled with or cooked in olive oil. You even have the option of having delicious raw vegetables for instance in a healthy salad. For a keto Mediterranean diet. The vegetables you select should be low in carbohydrate content, so avoid starchy vegetables like potatoes. Instead, you have a wide variety of good keto-friendly vegetables to choose from which have been a part of the Mediterranean diet for years together.

Some of the recommended vegetables in the Mediterranean diet are listed below:

Artichokes

You can enjoy the soft, deep and subtle flavors of this incredible green by steaming it. This vegetable is rich in magnesium, iron, vitamin C, and antioxidants, and it has prebiotic properties as well. So, this helps improve your gut's health.

Arugula

The peppery flavor and aroma of arugula adds a wonderful texture to a salad. This vegetable is rich in chlorophyll and helps to prevent DNA and liver damage caused by aflatoxins. Aflatoxins are certain harmful carcinogens that are produced by specific molds that grow in soil and decaying vegetables and grains.

Beets

Beets, also known as beetroots, are vegetables rich in manganese, folate, and iron, and are packed with essential minerals, vitamins and plant compounds with medicinal properties. Beets taste delicious and are extremely easy to add to your diet.

Cabbage

Cabbages are often overlooked although they are packed with nutrients and are rich in antioxidants that help prevent inflammation.

Brussels Sprouts

Brussels sprouts resemble a mini cabbage and are packed with nutrients, antioxidants and fiber.

Celery

Celery is a crispy and crunchy vegetable that is low in calories, rich in antioxidants, and aids in digestion.

Chicory
The chicory root is a food additive found in a variety of products, like in coffee and as a food additive. This root is rich in dietary fiber, which is soluble in insulin. Dietary fiber helps reduce the absorption of carbs and this in turn reduces the blood glucose and insulin levels. The reduction of these levels in helpful while fighting obesity and diabetes.

Cucumbers
Cucumber is a fruit. It is low in calories and has large amounts of water and dietary fiber, aiding in weight loss and increasing hydration.

Eggplant
Eggplants have a toothsome texture and very neutral flavor, making it very suitable for sauces quite nicely. This vegetable can also be used to mimic meat. It is a nutritional powerhouse with fiber and potassium. A concentrated compound in the skin called chlorogenic acid also has anti-viral and anti-cancer properties.

Fennel
Fennel is packed with copper, zinc, calcium, potassium, vitamin C, selenium, manganese, magnesium and iron. Fennel seeds are packed

with nutrients that assist in water retention and regulating blood pressure.

Mustard Greens

Mustard greens are loaded with nutrients that ward off diseases. They have a rich, peppery flavor and are so light in calories that you can eat as much as you want.

Mushrooms

Mushrooms are a type of fungi, and are rich in protein, fiber, and antioxidants.

Kale

Kale is one of the most nutritious leafy greens loaded with nutrients and antioxidants, and it can help lower cholesterol.

Leeks

Leeks are sweet and can be eaten cooked or raw. This vegetable has antimicrobial properties and is rich in antioxidants.

Bell Peppers

Peppers can be eaten in any way, such as fresh, ground, or roasted, and are rich sources of vitamin A, and vitamin C. They also contain folate, fiber, beta-carotene and some vitamin K. Red peppers contain lycopene and lutein, which aid infighting macular degeneration.

Christine Moore

These are many more vegetables available that you can choose from for your Keto-friendly Mediterranean meals. They can all be cooked or consumed in a variety of ways, keeping your meals appetizing and healthy. Other vegetables you can eat include turnips, zucchini, onions, radishes, peas, okra, broccoli, scallions, and spinach.

Chapter 8:
Keto Mediterranean Meats and Nuts

In this chapter, we will talk about Mediterranean foods in the form of fish, meats, nuts, and beans, that are keto friendly and can be a part of your diet. These are all foods that can easily be found and thus made a part of your meals. These foods have been consumed as a part of the daily diets of the people who live in the countries around the Mediterranean Sea and are their main source of protein. It is important to provide your body with some good protein even when you are trying to lose weight. It plays an important role in your body and prevents muscle wasting as well. As you read on you will understand why we recommend these foods and why they are an important part of your diet.

Let's first start with fish since they are the best source of protein in the Mediterranean diet, rather than other meats. Consumption of fish that is rich in omega-3 fats is considered one of the healthiest aspects of the Keto-Mediterranean diet. This includes fish like wild salmon, which is quite oily. A study published in the Nutrition Research journal in 2016 showed that overweight men or women who started consuming salmon a couple of times a week saw improvement in their blood fat profile.

The more fish is consumed, the better its health benefits. Consuming salmon aids in reducing triglycerides in the blood and increases HDL cholesterol levels. There is also a positive impact on lipoprotein molecule sizes, which is important as it helps to reduce the risk of coronary artery disease. A diet that includes salmon will be very good for the health of the heart. It is recommended to consume ocean fish or wild fish instead of farmed fish, if possible. The former contains more levels of omega-3 fatty acids that are beneficial for health. You also should be careful about consuming too much tuna or swordfish because these types of fish can contain high levels of mercury, that is very toxic when it builds up. A lot of people suffer from mercury toxicity due to over-consumption of these fish so you should consume them sparingly. The Keto-Mediterranean diet recommends fish as a part of your diet 2-3 times a week. Include fish that contain low levels of mercury such as sardines, salmon, flounder, shrimp, crab, lobster or cod. Limit the consumption of bluefish, tuna, Chilean sea bass, swordfish, halibut or grouper. These types of fish will increase oxidative stress in your body and reduce intracellular glutathione. To counter mercury toxicity, you can inquire about selenium supplements.

Some years ago, people started discouraging the consumption of nuts because these are high in fat; however, the Keto-Mediterranean diet prompts you to consume nuts in your diet for the very same reason and emphasizes that they are healthy. You should be careful and consume a limited amount, but there is no reason to cut them out of your diet completely. Nuts are healthy ingredients that can reduce the risk of cancer, cardiovascular diseases, as well as increase longevity. Studies were conducted to compare those who consumed a limited quantity of nuts every day to those who did not. The research showed that the ones who consumed nuts had a significantly lower risk of heart diseases. The European Journal of Nutrition also published a study that said walnuts, peanuts and other such nuts helped to reduce weight and prevention of obesity. This is because the nuts are very low in carbohydrates and rich in fiber.

Another study conducted and published in the New England Journal of Medicine stated that amongst people with a high risk of cardiovascular diseases, those who consumed a Mediterranean diet were at much lower risk, demonstrating that the diet actually reduces the chances of many illnesses, slows down the aging process and also increases life expectancy.

The following are some of the nuts, beans, legumes and seeds, and seafood that can be included in the Ketogenic Mediterranean diet. You will also learn of some of their benefits and why you should consume them.

Almonds

They are a rich source of vitamin E, healthy fats, protein and other minerals. Almonds are considered helpful in lowering blood sugar levels, blood pressure and high cholesterol. They also aid in reducing cravings and thus promote weight loss. They contain many bioactive molecules that can help in the prevention of cardiovascular diseases.

Cashews

A lot of people avoid this nut because they think it will make them fat; however, cashews can have a lot of health benefits and should be added to your diet in a limited quantity. They are high in fat and are also a good source of vitamin E and minerals like zinc and magnesium. They also aid in boosting the immune system and have anti-cancerous properties.

Hazelnuts

Hazelnuts are very common in the region of Italy and can be eaten as snacks, used in sauces, or added on as a garnish to your dish. They contain a lot of monounsaturated fat and are a good source of vitamin E, folate, protein, calcium and fiber. It also contains arginine, which is beneficial for the blood vessels.

Pistachios

Pistachios are very rich in nutrient and taste delicious. They aid in digestion and help to control diabetes. Pistachios are considered helpful in the management of weight and reduce bad LDL cholesterol levels. They are rich in antioxidants and contribute to skin hydration. They can also reduce the risk of macular disease related to age.

Walnuts

They contain MUFA and PUFA, which are the healthy fats your diet needs. They are a super source of omega-3 fatty acids, as well as iron, selenium, zinc and calcium. They promote a healthy gut and help lower blood pressure. They are also used in the management of Type 2 Diabetes and reduce inflammation.

Pine Nuts

They contribute to good heart health and are a great source of monounsaturated fatty acids. Pine nuts can help lower LDL and the risk of heart attacks. They have a light taste and texture that makes them a great ingredient in salads.

Split Peas

They provide vitamin K, which promotes the heart as well as bone health. They also contain thiamine and fiber, which helps in blood sugar management and supporting brain health. They are very rich sources of minerals for your diet.

Kidney Beans

Kidney beans are a power-packed source of proteins and minerals. They lower cholesterol levels and are a good ingredient for people with diabetes. They are considered helpful in losing weight and promote good colon health. They have detoxifying properties and boost energy. Kidney beans are also said to aid in the prevention of hypertension and memory retention.

Fava Beans

These beans are dense with nutrition and contain no saturated fat. They help in the treatment of Parkinson's disease symptoms and reduce symptoms of anemia too. They contain a high amount of thiamine, vitamin B6 and K, copper, magnesium and selenium. They also boost the immune system and can help in the prevention of congenital disabilities.

Sesame Seeds

They are rich in polyunsaturated fatty acids as well as omega-3 fatty acids. They are good for skin and hair health. They also boost energy levels and promote bone health. The magnesium content in sesame seeds is considered helpful in preventing hypertension.

Chickpeas

If you eat them daily, chickpeas provide protein, folate, calcium, iron and zinc. They are also a good source of soluble and insoluble fibers that will keep you full for longer periods. Chickpeas also have phytate and phytosterols and can help manage diabetes or reducing the risk of heart disease or colon cancer.

Lentils

They are very low in calories and are a great source of iron, folate and protein. They have a high content of polyphenols that promote good health and reduce the risk of heart diseases. The complex carbs in lentils help to boost metabolism and aid the process of burning fats. The fiber in lentils reduces cholesterol levels in the blood.

The following are some of the fish and meats that you should include in your diet. You can eat them for lunch or dinner a couple of times a week. Try to consume more of fish than meat, as they are a good source of omega-3 fatty acids that will benefit your heart. People in the Mediterranean countries tend to eat meat in very small portions, and more often than naught prefer lean cuts. Poultry is one of the better sources of lean protein since it does not have the high amount of saturated fats that can be found in some red meats.

Abalone

Abalones can be eaten raw or cooked, taste great either way. They are a great source of vital nutrients and are especially beneficial for eye and skin health. They are low in fat and provide omega-3 fatty acids to your diet.

Clams

Clams are a nutritious food with many health benefits. You get lean protein, minerals and vitamins along with omega-3 fatty acids. They also aid in sexual health, and they may have anti-cancer properties. They are very low in carbs and calories, so they also aid in weight loss.

Crab

Crab has very little fat, is low in calories, and tastes great. It is free of carbohydrates and aids in building muscle while losing weight. It is considered healthy for the diet of expectant mothers and is a good source of riboflavin and selenium.

Mackerel

Mackerel is an oily fish that is rich in omega-3 fatty acids, helping to reduce inflammation and the risk of cardiovascular diseases, cancer and arthritis. It is also a good source of lean protein. The calcium in it also aids in burning fat and maintaining bone health.

Oyster

Oysters are aphrodisiacs and are good for sexual health. They are very low in calories, fats and carbohydrates. They are a great source of protein and keep you satiated after a meal. They are also a good source of vitamin A, vitamin E and minerals like iron, calcium and selenium.

Salmon

Salmon is one of the best sources of omega-3 fatty acids and protein in the diet. It also contains the antioxidant astaxanthin, which benefits your health. It is very dense in nutrients and promotes heart health.

Shrimp

Shrimp provides protein, selenium and niacin. They are low in calories and help in weight loss. They promote bone strength, mental health and cardiovascular health. They are also good for the eyes.

Sea Bass

Sea bass is a great source of protein and selenium and is very low in calories. The high level of omega-3 fatty acids makes it healthy, especially aiding in eye health. It is also a source of vitamin B12 and vitamin B6.

Flounder

Flounder is a heart-healthy ingredient in your diet and provides many essential nutrients.

Tilapia

Tilapia contains very little fat or calories and aids in weight loss. It also protects the body from symptoms of aging, reduces cholesterol and triglycerides and contains no carbohydrates.

Yellowtail

Yellowtail is a delicacy that is rich and fatty and a great source of omega-3 fatty acids. It is said to help in the treatment of depression and lifts the mood. It also aids in lowering blood pressure and reducing inflammation during arthritis.

Squid

It contains vitamins and minerals like vitamin B12, iron, copper and potassium. It promotes healthy blood cells and boosts the immune system. It can also aid in reducing levels of bad cholesterol or LDL.

Sardines

Sardines are good for the heart and a great source of vitamin B12. The mercury content is also minimal, and they are also high in vitamin D.

Beef
They are a great source of niacin, riboflavin and vitamin B6. The protein from beef helps to build bone strength and muscle growth. The selenium in beef supports the immune system.

Chicken
Chicken is a good source of low-fat protein, and it contributes to muscle growth and development. It is also a good source of vitamin B6, niacin and selenium. The chicken breast is considered useful in controlling homocysteine levels, which helps to reduce the risk of heart diseases.

Duck
The monounsaturated fat found in duck helps to reduce LDL and increasing HDL. It is a good source of niacin, riboflavin, thiamine, zinc and iron. It supports cardiovascular health and is also rich in vitamin B6.

Goat
The vitamin B in goat meat helps to burn fat in the body. It contains a lot of lean protein and very little saturated fat, which aids in weight loss. The selenium and choline content of this meat help to prevent cancer. It is leaner than meat from beef, pork or chicken.

Lamb

Lamb is a good source of protein that is of high quality and contains vitamins and minerals. The nutrients of this meat promote growth and development of muscles. It is also helpful in maintaining healthy levels of cholesterol and is a good source of selenium.

Guinea Fowl

Guinea fowl has low levels of cholesterol and fats and is a healthy choice for your meal. The eggs are also healthy and contain vitamin E, vitamin D3 and vitamin A. The meat of the fowl supports heart health and boosts mental health.

Another great source of high-quality protein is eggs. They are a very common part of the Mediterranean diet and are especially good for people who don't consume any meat. You can opt for chicken eggs, duck eggs or even quail eggs.

Chapter 9:
Keto-Mediterranean Fruits and Dairy Products

Fruits are healthy foods that should be part of your diet, consumed whole and fresh in order to obtain the maximum nutritional benefit from them. However, processed fruit juices are not as beneficial since they are filled with added sugar and preservatives. Unlike vegetables, however, you will need to control your fruit portions due to the higher content of carbohydrates. As mentioned earlier, fruits like mangoes and bananas are rich in natural sugar and should be limited.

Some of the recommended Keto-Mediterranean fruit are listed below along with their health benefits:

Apple
Apples contain flavonoids, which are antioxidants that can help to reduce the risk of diabetes and asthma. They can also help cleanse the oral cavity. The skin of the apple should not be peeled since it contains most of the vitamins.

Apricot

Apricots are a great source of Vitamin A, which promotes eye health. They provide iron to fight anemia and have pectin, which treats constipation. They are diet-friendly and benefit the skin and bone health. For pregnant women, apricots are considered helpful and nutritious.

Cherry

Cherries are a popular fruit of many varieties. The sour variety contains a better nutritional profile compared to the sweeter cherries. They contain vitamin A, vitamin C, potassium, copper and manganese.

Dates

Dates are very nutritious and high in fiber content. They contain antioxidants, help to promote brain health and are also a great natural sweetener. The fruit can also aid in natural labor. They also contain various vitamins and minerals.

Grapes

Grapes are packed with vitamin C and vitamin K. and antioxidants, which can protect against chronic disease. Resveratrol in grapes is a key nutrient that can benefit your body. Grapes can also decrease levels of blood sugar in the body and protect from Type 2 Diabetes.

Cucumbers

Cucumber is a fruit. It is low in calories and has large amounts of water and dietary fiber, aiding in weight loss and increasing hydration.

Melon

Melons contain heart-supporting elements like vitamin C, fiber, potassium and choline. The potassium helps to reduce blood pressure.

Olives

Olives have great antioxidant properties that reduce the risk of heart diseases, cancer, and return blood cholesterol and blood pressure to a normal level. Olives are also said to benefit bone health and boost iron intake in the body.

Orange

A single orange can provide you with a variety of vitamins and minerals. It is a rich source of vitamin C and can significantly reduce the risk of ischemic stroke in women. It also helps to prevent damage to skin and lowers bad cholesterol or high blood sugar.

Pomegranate

This fruit is very rich in vitamin C and potassium. It is also a good source of fiber. This fruit helps in digestion and protection against heart disease, arthritis and Alzheimer's.

Strawberry

Strawberries are a very rich source of antioxidants and protect against free radicals. It is good for weight management and helps to reduce blood sugar regulation. This fruit also has anti-microbial properties and is good for the heart and immune system.

Clementine

Clementine's are rich in nutrients that are vital for health. They contain a lot of calcium, potassium, phosphorus and magnesium. They provide vitamin C and folate. Clementine's promote good vision and is beneficial for the skin and digestive system.

Blueberry

Blueberries are quite low in carbohydrates and are rich in polyphenols that are good for health. They also contain vitamin C, vitamin E, vitamin B6, vitamin K and manganese.

Blackberry

They are a good source of vitamin C and contain a relatively low amount of sugar compared to other fruit. They also provide manganese, vitamin K and vitamin E.

Peach

Peaches contain nutrients and vitamins like vitamin E, vitamin A and vitamin C. Peaches are low in calories and boost metabolism. The catechins in peaches help to burn calories and aid in weight loss.

Fig

This fruit is rich in fiber, and this keeps you full for a long time. It also aids in relieving constipation. Figs are a good source of vitamin A, vitamin B1 and vitamin B2. They can also aid in lowering blood sugar and blood cholesterol levels. The calcium content of a fig helps to prevent osteoporosis.

Avocados

They are a good source of Vitamin E and folate. Avocados contain monounsaturated fats that aid in lowering bad cholesterol levels. The cold -pressed oil obtained from this fruit is nearly as healthy as olive oil. It is also a very versatile fruit and can be used in many different dishes.

Tangerine

They provide a lot of nutrients like potassium and thiamine to the body. They are a low-calorie fruit that contain more vitamin A than almost any other fruit. The high content of fiber relieves constipation, and it also aids in iron absorption.

Tomato

Tomatoes are not native to the Mediterranean but are always found in Mediterranean kitchens. They are packed with lycopene, which is an antioxidant that protects the heart. They also contain a lot of vitamin C and add flavor to all kinds of dishes.

Pear

This fruit is full of fiber and is beneficial for skin health. It is also beneficial in treating diverticulosis and aids in preventing cardiovascular diseases. Pears are a detoxifying fruit and aid in digestion. They are a good source of vitamin C.

The following are some of the dairy products that will benefit your Ketogenic Mediterranean diet process and help you stay healthy while losing weight.

Brie

The protein found in Brie can provide your body with every amino acid it requires. This cheese has lower fat and calorie content than other cheeses. It is also lower in carbohydrate content. Every ounce of Brie has about 6 grams of protein and 8 grams of fat.

Feta

Feta cheese is usually made with milk from sheep or goats. It has a good amount of vitamin B and calcium. It also has bacteria that are beneficial for gut health. Due to the high saturated fat and sodium content, you should consume this cheese carefully. It is considered one of the best cheeses in a diet meant for weight loss.

Chevre

Chevre is a goat milk cheese that provides healthy fats to the body. It also provides probiotic bacteria and is easier to digest than some other cheeses. It aids in reducing hunger cravings and is a good source of calcium and protein.

Haloumi

It is considered a healthy cheese that is very low in carbohydrate content. It is naturally salty and is a good option for the vegetarian diet.

Pecorino

It is a good source of calcium, potassium and protein. It is usually used as an alternative for Parmesan cheese and has a sharper taste, so a little is usually enough.

Yogurt

Yogurts are usually high in protein, calcium, probiotics and vitamins. They aid in maintaining bone health and can protect from osteoporosis. Yogurt aids in the digestive process and is a good source of protein in a diet meant for weight loss.

Ricotta

Ricotta cheese has a texture that is like cottage cheese, although it is lighter. It can provide a lot of calcium and protein in even a small amount. This cheese is low in sodium content and higher in phosphorous and vitamin content. It is also a good source of omega fatty acids.

Manchego

This cheese is commonly consumed in Spain, is a very good source of protein and can be eaten even if you have high cholesterol. It provides a lot of calcium, which ensures good bone health and is recommended for pregnant women, children and the elderly. It is also a lactose-free cheese and works as a laxative too.

The following are the best oils for the Keto-Mediterranean diet:

Olive Oil

When it comes to oils, your best bet is olive oil. We have already mentioned in previous chapters how this oil is beneficial to your health. Olives or olive oil is quite central to the diet of the Mediterranean region. You can opt to have whole olives in your diet or use the oil for cooking or flavoring your food. Olive oil is the main dietary fat source that is used in cooking and baking or in dressings on salads and vegetables. The highest amount of health-promoting fats can be found in extra virgin olive oil, which will also provide you with a lot of phytonutrients and many other micronutrients that are important for your body.

Avocado oil

It is very rich in oleic acid that is a healthy fat. It helps to reduce bad cholesterol and aids in improving heart health. This oil has a high amount of lutein that is an antioxidant that benefits eye health. It also enhances nutrient absorption in the body and can improve the skin. It can also help to reduce symptoms of arthritis and gum disease.

Canola Oil

Canola oil is a healthy cooking oil that contains omega-3 fatty acids as well as omega 6 fatty acids. The reduced saturated fat in this oil helps to reduce cholesterol. It is also rich in vitamin E and vitamin K, which aid in maintaining healthy skin and reducing signs of aging like wrinkles and blemishes.

From all the information given above, you can understand why we recommend these food items and ingredients in your diet. They are all keto-friendly, and are already a part of the Mediterranean diet, aiding in overall wellbeing while helping you to

Chapter 10:
Finding Your Carb Sweet Spot

The Ketogenic Mediterranean diet is a very low carb diet but not one that eliminates carbohydrates. In the limited quantity of carbohydrates that are allowed in the diet, it is important to consider what you should eat. To enjoy the best benefits of this diet, you should include carbs that will still let your body stay in the state of ketosis to keep burning fats successfully. For this, you must find a way to benefit from the carbohydrates in your diet without suffering any of the negative impacts.

Carbohydrates have their benefits. They help to increase leptin levels, improve libido, increase metabolism and increase anabolism; however, we rarely reap these benefits because it is easy to consume too many carbohydrates and then you are just impacted by the negative aspect. Eating too much carbohydrate loaded food and at the wrong time will only lead to excessive body weight. If you completely cut them off, then you will miss out on the performance-enhancing benefit of carbs. So, the question is how to find the carb sweet spot while maintaining ketosis in the Ketogenic Mediterranean diet.

The carbohydrate-limiting factor can be confusing. You might be wondering what you can or cannot eat in the form of carbs and how can you eat carbs without affecting ketosis in your body. If you follow the Mediterranean food guide while on the keto diet, you don't really have to worry about the bad carb or good carb options. Most of your food will be healthy on this diet anyway. Occasionally eating a little bit of a bad carb might work as a treat for you too.

In the ketogenic diet, it is recommended to eat complex carbohydrate foods and avoid simple carbohydrates. Complex carbohydrates include unrefined whole grain bread, unrefined brown rice, beans, chickpeas, carrots and leafy greens. Simple carbohydrates include white bread, white rice, processed cereals and refined pasta, candy, and fruit juices. You should limit the low carb foods to sources such as berries and leafy greens, which will allow you to stay in the limit of daily carb consumption while getting enough fiber and micronutrients. You need to kick off the habit of consuming refined grains, sugar and such simple carbohydrates that will compromise the process of ketosis.

The best options that will help you stay healthy are complex carbohydrate sources like eggplant, broccoli, and asparagus. Potatoes are a bad carb that you need to avoid since a single large potato will cross your daily carb limit quite easily. When you are on a keto diet, you should stick to unrefined complex carbs that will help to lower your blood glucose levels. This way you won't have to depend on any glucose supporting supplements.

The complex carbs will provide enough energy to keep your body functioning and healthy. The sources we recommended in this diet will also support a healthy gut and provide you with essential micronutrients.

To determine how much carbohydrate the body will need without gaining weight, you must keep a few factors in mind.

Your body type plays a role in determining its own ability to handle any carbohydrates. Ectomorphs are more capable of consuming carbs than their counterparts. Thus, the former should consume more compared to the latter.

The body fat to muscle ratio in a person will help to determine how tolerant his or her body is with carbs. People who have higher muscle mass and lesser body fat are more tolerant and can consume more carbohydrates. Those with higher fats and less muscle tend to store fat and should consume fewer carbohydrates.

The amount of carbs a person requires also depends on their activity levels. The more energy they burn, the more carbs they need. The more sedentary their lifestyle, the fewer carbs they require.

These factors will give you an idea about how many carbs you should consume in your diet, and you can adjust the numbers accordingly. Ultimately you must remember that the Ketogenic Mediterranean diet is very low in carbohydrates and only requires the minimum essential amount of this macronutrient.

Some dietitians also recommend that the individual increase their awareness of what the body needs. If you feel that you had a high-performance day and your body needs a little extra carbohydrate, then it is okay to provide it with the carbs in moderation. If you feel that you had a very sedentary day with barely any physical activity, then you probably don't require any at all.

On days that you skip your regular workout, you can also afford to skip your carbohydrate dose. Your body is the best guide that you should listen to. Listen to common sense and fight any unhealthy cravings at the beginning of your diet and later you should listen to your body and eat accordingly. For instance, some people find it healthier to eat three meals in one day while others eat smaller portions throughout the day. It can differ from person to person, and there is no single right or wrong way. It takes time to develop body awareness and can be very easy to mix up signals sent by the body. Take the time to learn and get to recognize its needs.

In the ketogenic diet, the usual carb limit is total carbs of 35 grams and net carbs of 25 grams; however, there is no specific number that the Ketogenic Mediterranean diet recommends. You shouldn't punish yourself for consuming some fruit in the evening. Each person has a different carb limit that they should set. This limit can differ from person to person, and even for that individual, it can be different on any given day.

Achieving ketosis will depend on many other factors and not just the carbohydrate intake of that day. There are people whose bodies kick into ketosis only when carbs are below 35 grams while others can consume more and still burn fat. This can make it challenging to determine what your limit is. Until you figure it out, you can use the general ketogenic diet limit for carbs that we mentioned earlier. It is found to be effective for most people who started on this diet and should work for you too. A lot of people also found that reducing the carbs to 20 grams helps to speed up ketosis in the body. It can help to maintain constant ketosis and losing weight.

The following are carbohydrate sources that you should and should not eat to maintain ketosis:

- Don't eat wheat, rice, corn or any such grains that are loaded with carbs.
- Avoid honey, maple syrup and other such sugar sources.
- Avoid fruits like bananas that are rich in sugar carbs.
- Don't eat potatoes and yams.

- Eat a moderate quantity of berries because they contain fewer carbs than other fruit and are also a powerhouse of antioxidants.
- Add avocados to your diet, as they are low in carbs, high in fat and fiber and are great for keto.
- Eat more lean meats like poultry and fish.
- Eat leafy greens that have a very little digestible fat and mostly contain fiber and water.
- Eat high-fat dairy like hard cheeses and fatty creams.
- Eat macadamia nuts, walnut and sunflower seeds. They are low in carbs but high in fiber and fat.
- Use coconut oil, avocado oil and canola oil.

You must understand that everyone has a different carb sweet spot for ketosis. We have given you the general limit for carbs in your diet, but it may not work for certain people and it might stop working at a certain point in your diet as well. If this happens, you should consider some other factors that will then contribute to determining the limit and your ketosis.

The process of keto-adaptation changes your body's ketone burning ability and your carb limit. Every person's body can burn ketones for energy. During keto-adaptation, mitochondria in the body starts working more efficiently and replicates. They then provide other cells with the ability to burn ketones for fuel instead of using sugar. This kind of adaptation helps the body to enter ketosis quickly. The more adapted you get to the ketogenic diet, the more carbs you can consume while maintaining ketosis over time.

If you want to take advantage of this adaptation, you should maintain the diet strictly for at least four to six months. During this period don't make any changes to the given plan and follow it blindly. You shouldn't increase your carbohydrate intake from 35 grams during the keto-adaptation period so that there is constant ketosis and your cells get used to the process. It is the only way you can reap the adaptation benefits later.

Another factor that is important to boost ketosis is exercise. A lot of people try to avoid this aspect and so they don't reap the total benefits of the ketogenic diet. It is for this reason that we said that adapting to the Mediterranean lifestyle would help to reap more benefit from the ketogenic diet too.

The people of that region are quite proactive in exercising and maintaining fitness and thus have a lower incidence of obesity. If you start the right type of exercise, it can help you to achieve ketosis even faster and boost the level of ketones in your body. If you want a rapid onset of ketosis, you should give serious consideration to high-intensity training. It will aid in depleting the stored glycogen in your body. Low-intensity training can be used to encourage more fat-burning.

When you are beginning the Ketogenic Mediterranean diet, focus first on depleting the storage of glycogen. This will push the body into ketosis faster. You can do this by practicing an hour of some high-intensity exercise in the morning like heavyweights, cross fit, and HIIT. When the workout is complete, you should give your body time to recover. Make sure you rehydrate and take some mineral supplements. Also, avoid eating anything till mealtime.

When the glycogen level in your body is depleted, low-intensity training will help to increase ketones and burning fat. This can be done by about half an hour of brisk walking or cycling before breakfast. If you do all this at the right time every day, it will help you achieve ketosis quite quickly. You will also be able to increase the carbohydrate limit in your diet without compromising on your ketone levels. You should also remember not to over-do high-intensity exercise as it can overwhelm your body and impair the ketosis ability of your body.

Stress is another important factor to consider since it can impair the ability of your body to carry out ketosis and will decrease your carbohydrate intake limit in the diet. The stress hormone levels increase in people who suffer from anxiety or stress on a regular basis. Cortisol is one of the stress hormones released during stress, and it increases gluconeogenesis in the body, which in turn decreases insulin sensitivity in the body. This results in increased blood sugar for a longer period, and thus the body does not require ketone production. You must remember that cortisol is not the enemy since it is a hormone that helps in different situations. There will be an issue if your body is incapable of producing cortisol.

The problem is stress in the process of ketosis and your diet. There are certain stressors that you need to avoid like worrying about the future or overwhelming yourself with work. A lot of people get stressed by thinking too much about past mistakes instead of moving on. Eating too little or exercising too much will also stress your body and mind. It is important to pace yourself, rest and give your body time to recover. This way you can avoid stress and alleviate the levels of stress hormones that limit the body's ketone production abilities. Stress will prevent you from losing weight and affect your ability to maintain muscle mass too. You need to avoid all such factors while you are on the Ketogenic Mediterranean diet if you want to see real results and stay healthy. Certain strategies will help you reduce stress and maintain ketosis. This includes eating the right quantity of calories in your diet, avoiding excessive exercise, improving the sleep cycle and practicing meditation. Meditation is considered very helpful in reducing stress and decreasing cortisol levels in the body.

Protein intake is also a factor that can block ketosis in your body. If your diet consists of too much protein, it floods the body with amino acids. In response to this, insulin will be released, and the body gets the signal that enough energy is available in the form of the amino acids. Due to this, they don't kickstart the process of ketosis and fat burning for energy. Thus, you can see that high protein meals can prevent ketosis in the body or cause a stall at some point. You shouldn't just focus on restricting carbohydrates during your diet but also on maintaining the right level of all the macros. The right balance in your diet will make a big difference.

The 35-gram total carb limit is generally ideal for everyone at least in the first few months of the ketogenic diet. It is important to consider the factors we mentioned like your stress level, exercise, and protein intake. They will all help in determining if your carb limit should be reduced or increased to improve the process of ketosis in your body. Finding your carb limit can be more complex than you might expect so try not to experiment too much in the beginning.

When you want to find your carb limit, certain steps will help. Keep track of your ketones with the help of a blood ketone meter. Increase your intake of carbs and keep tracking the ketone levels over time. First, give your body time to establish ketosis for some time by using the 35-gram limit. Then, after a while, increase your limit by 5 grams each day. These carbs should still be healthy for you and not some candies or simple sugars. Such simple carbs will rapidly increase your insulin levels and kick you out of ketosis. Increasing complex carbs from plant-based sources will help. Take the ketone measurement in your blood at the same time every single day. This will help you in seeing if the increased carbohydrates decreased your blood ketone level.

After increasing the limit, if you see that the ketone level has not decreased, you can increase the limit a little more after time. Repeat the tracking process again and decrease the carb limit of you see that the ketone level decrease. You should always aim to maintain a level of ketosis according to the weight goal that you have set. For those who want to lose significant weight, it should be in a state of deep ketosis with 1.5 mmol/L to 3.0 mmol/L. Blood ketone meters are the only way to determine the level of ketosis accurately. During the first couple of days of the ketogenic diet, most people will find that they are in a state of light ketosis. Deep ketosis kicks in only after a couple of weeks. The tips in this chapter aim to help you kick in ketosis even more rapidly. While you are maintaining the limit of 35 grams of carbs, monitor your progress. If it is working well and helping you lose enough weight, there is no reason to increase or decrease your limit until you reach your goal or hit a weight stall. Experimenting too much for no reason will only complicate the process for you.

Your carb limit will depend on factors like sleep and activity that we discussed earlier. If you are exercising a little extra today, you can add a few extra grams of carbohydrate for that day without guilt. It takes time, patience and persistence to find the carb limit for ketosis in your body. You must track the changes in your body and life to get the best results while you follow the Ketogenic Mediterranean diet.

For athletes or high-intensity trainers, carbohydrates can play a major role. They cannot always afford to consume too few carbs in their diet. For beginners in high-intensity training, the targeted ketogenic version of the diet is recommended. In this case, the person can consume an extra 10-20 grams of carbs that are easily digestible. This should be done about half an hour before they exercise. This is only for beginners and not for athletes and regular trainers. These people might require the cyclical version of the ketogenic diet. This version involves a couple of days of increased carb followed by the ketogenic regime the rest of the week. It helps combine ketosis with carbohydrates for improving the athlete's strength and performance. They need to deplete their glycogen stores before they start the refeeding cycle.

Ketone boosting supplements are another factor that you can consider for boosting ketosis in your body. One is ketone salt, which is a powder containing ketone bodies with minerals. Usually, they contain calcium, potassium, magnesium or sodium and these are bound with acetoacetate or beta-hydroxybutyrate.

Consumption of ketone salts helps to significantly increase ketone levels without the waiting period required in the standard diet. But there are studies that show that these ketone salts can impair the body's ability to maintaining ketosis in the long term. The salts should not be used as a replacement for the limit of carbs either.

The standard ketogenic diet is much more beneficial in the long run and is a healthier option too. You can consider certain ketone salts if you suffer from some mineral deficiency that it can act as a supplement for. MCT oil is the other supplement used in ketosis. MCT stands for medium chain triglycerides, and these can be broken down in the liver to ketone bodies. This happens whether the body has entered ketosis. They are saturated fats unlike any other type of saturated fat. They will help to skip the part of fat digestion and are directly converted into ketone bodies in the liver regardless of following the ketogenic diet.

In natural form, these are found in coconuts, but the easiest way is to take them in the form of the MCT oil supplement. The best supplement is one that contains caprylic acid. This MCT is known to get digested and converted to ketones faster than other types. You must remember that none of the ketone boosting supplements will benefit you like the actual ketogenic diet and they should only be used as a last resort or temporarily.

Everyone will not get the same result from the same carb limit. The ketone levels in your body will depend on the level of activity you perform, the amount of protein you consume, your stress levels and your keto-adaptation period. For this reason, some people thrive on a higher intake of carbohydrates while others require less. Supplements will help you to a certain extent, but the Ketogenic Mediterranean diet is your best bet for a healthy process of weight loss. As you keep reading, you will also learn about how intermittent fasting will aid this process.

Christine Moore

Chapter 11:
Intermittent Fasting

The intermittent fasting diet is one of the most popular fitness and health trends in the world. People use this method to improve their health, change their lifestyles and lose weight. Many studies talk about the powerful effects that this lifestyle has on a person's brain and body. Some studies also show that this lifestyle can help you live a longer life. We will cover some of the basics of intermittent fasting in this chapter.

Intermittent fasting is an eating pattern where you shift between periods of eating and fasting. This pattern does not specify which food you should eat but tells you when you should be consuming those foods. Therefore, one cannot use the conventional term "diet" to describe this eating. As mentioned earlier, this is an eating pattern. Some methods of intermittent fasting involve a sixteen-hour fast or a 24-hour fast at least twice a week.

Throughout human evolution, human beings have practiced fasting. Our ancestors did not have refrigerators, grocery stores or food available throughout the year. There were times when they did not find any food that they could eat. As a result, human beings could survive and function without any food for a long period. Fasting is considered more natural when compared to consuming at least four meals a day. Some people also fast for spiritual or religious reasons, and many religions like Islam, Hinduism, Judaism, Christianity and Buddhism promote fasting.

Intermittent Fasting Methods

You can follow different eating patterns if you choose to follow the intermittent fasting lifestyle. Each of these patterns will involve splitting the week or day into fasting and eating periods. You either eat nothing or very little during the fasting period. The most popular methods of intermittent fasting are:

Eat-Stop-Eat

In this method, you will need to fast for at least twenty-four hours either once or twice a week. For example, you could skip dinner tonight and not eat any food until dinner the following night.

The 16/8 Method

The 16/8 method, also known as the Lean Gains protocol, requires you to skip breakfast every day and restrict the eating period to eight hours only. You can eat between 1 PM and 9 PM or any other period depending on your convenience. You will then need to fast for sixteen hours.

The 5:2 Diet

In this method, you will normally eat on five days of the week but consume only 600 calories on two non-consecutive days.

These methods will help you lose weight, if you do not consume more calories than needed during the eating period. People prefer the 16/8 method since that is the easiest method to stick to, and it is sustainable.

Alternate Day Fasting

As the name suggests, in this fasting you only fast on alternate days. There are variations of this method. In some of the variations, you can consume 500 calories on alternate days while on others you are asked to follow a strict fast and only drink water. The benefits of this diet are the same as those of any other type of intermittent fasting. A strict diet can be overwhelming for a beginner, so you can modify this diet to suit your needs. However, you should be prepared to overcome pangs of hunger on some days.

Skipping Meals Spontaneously

As the name suggests, there is no plan for this diet. You can reap the benefits of the intermittent fasting diet without having to plan elaborate meals. This is a simple variation to follow since you only need to skip meals occasionally. When you are not hungry or are occupied with some work, you can skip a meal since you will not be thinking about food. People do not have to eat every two hours, and your body will not starve if you do not give it food every two hours. The human body has been designed in a way to help you go without food for a long period. It is all right to miss two meals occasionally since it gives your body the opportunity to remove any toxins. So, if you are not hungry, you can skip the meal.

Every variation of intermittent fasting is effective, and it would be best for you to choose a variation that works best for you.

How Does Intermittent Fasting Affect Your Cells and Hormones?

Your body goes through several changes at the molecular and cellular levels when you fast. For instance, your body will adjust to all the hormone levels and make use of the stored fat in the body to produce energy. Your cells will also begin to repair and alter your genes. Let us look at some changes that will occur in your body when you fast.

Human Growth Hormone

The growth hormone levels will skyrocket. This helps you lose weight, shed fat and gain muscle mass.

Insulin

The levels of insulin in your blood will drop rapidly, and your body's sensitivity to insulin will improve. Your body can access the stored body fat easily if the levels of insulin are low.

Cellular Repair

When your body is in the fasting state, your cells will begin the repair process. This means that the cells will remove or digest dysfunctional and old proteins that develop in the cells. This process is called autophagy.

Gene Expression

Intermittent fasting will lead to some changes in the functions of genes that are associated with your immunity and longevity.

These changes in cell function, gene expression and hormone levels are the factors responsible for the health benefits of this eating pattern.

A Powerful Weight Loss Tool

Most people choose the intermittent fasting eating pattern to lose weight. When you reduce the number of meals you consume every day, you will automatically reduce your caloric intake. As mentioned earlier, the changes in the hormones aid in weight loss. In addition to this, intermittent fasting also helps to increase the quantity of noradrenaline or norepinephrine, the fat-burning hormone.

Your metabolic rate may increase between 3.6-14% because of the changes in your hormones. Since you will consume fewer calories and burn more calories, you will lose weight since the calorie equation will change.

Many studies show that intermittent fasting is an easy way to lose weight. A study showed that this eating pattern would help a person lose at least 3-8% of their weight in 24 weeks. This is a significant amount of loss, which is more than any other weight loss method. In the same study, people also lost at least 7% of their waist circumference which indicates that intermittent fasting helps to burn belly fat which accumulates around your organs and leads to numerous diseases. You should, however, keep in mind that intermittent fasting is successful since it ensures that you consume fewer calories. If you binge or eat large quantities of food during your eating periods, you will not lose any weight.

Health Benefits

There are many studies conducted on intermittent fasting using both animals and human beings as subjects. These studies show that intermittent fasting helps to improve the health of your brain and body, and aid in weight loss. Let us look at some of the benefits of intermittent fasting.

Weight Loss

As mentioned earlier, intermittent fasting will help you lose belly fat and weight, and you don't have to restrict your caloric intake consciously.

Insulin Resistance

Through intermittent fasting, one can overcome insulin resistance. This helps to reduce the level of blood sugar by at least 6%. This will protect your body against Type 2 Diabetes.

Inflammation

Studies show that intermittent fasting reduces the symptoms of inflammation, thereby reducing the risk of developing numerous chronic diseases.

Heart Health

Intermittent fasting will reduce bad cholesterol, blood sugar, inflammatory markers, insulin resistance and blood triglycerides, thereby reducing the probability of developing heart diseases.

Cancer

Many animal studies suggest that the intermittent fasting eating pattern helps to prevent the growth of cancerous cells.

Brain Health

The brain hormone, BDNF, is released in large quantities when you follow the intermittent fasting diet. This hormone will aid in the growth of new cells in the brain and may prevent the development of Alzheimer's.

Anti-Aging

Studies conducted on rats showed that intermittent fasting extends lifespan. This study showed that rats that were fasting lived at least 36-83% longer than rats that did not fast.

You should keep in mind that further research must be conducted to understand the benefits of intermittent fasting. The studies that have been conducted were short-term, small or conducted on animals. Some questions about how intermittent fasting affects human beings still need to be answered.

Makes Your Lifestyle Simpler

It is simple to eat healthy, but it is hard to maintain it. The main obstacle is the work you will need to put in to cooking healthy meals. You will need to plan your meals and procure your ingredients in advance. Intermittent fasting will make things easier since you do not have too many dishes to cook since you will be consuming fewer meals overall. You will also have fewer dishes to clean. It is for this reason that people who look for life-hacks follow the intermittent fasting diet. This diet will simplify your life and improve your health.

Who Should Avoid or Be Careful?

Not everyone can follow intermittent fasting or adopt this eating pattern as their lifestyle. If you are underweight or have an eating disorder, you should speak to your physician before you adopt this eating pattern. In some cases, this eating pattern is downright harmful.

Should Women Fast?

Some studies state that intermittent fasting is not as beneficial for women when compared to men. For instance, a study showed that intermittent fasting helped to improve insulin sensitivity in men and worsened the control of blood sugar in women.

According to some studies, intermittent fasting is not as beneficial for women when compared to men. Human studies are currently unavailable on this topic, and most studies have been conducted on rats. Studies showed that intermittent fasting could lead to infertility or missed menstrual cycles in female rats.

Some women reported that their menstrual period stopped when they adopted the intermittent fasting eating pattern. The menstrual cycle went back to normal when they began to eat normally. It is for this reason that women should be extremely careful when they adopt the intermittent fasting eating method. Women should follow a separate guideline, and ease into the practice slowly. They should stop immediately if they have any issues with menstruation. If you have any issues with fertility or are trying to conceive, you should avoid this eating pattern.

Side Effects and Safety

One of the main side effects of intermittent fasting is hunger. You will also feel weak until your body can handle the decreased quantity of glucose. There is a possibility that your brain may not perform as well as it used to until it adapts. As mentioned earlier, this is only temporary since it will take your body some time to adapt to the new schedule.

If you suffer from any medical conditions, you should check with your physician before you follow this eating pattern. This is especially important if you:

- Have trouble with the regulation of blood sugar

- Have diabetes

- Are on certain medications

- Have suffered from eating disorders in the past

- Have low blood pressure

- Are underweight

- Are pregnant or breastfeeding

- Are a woman who has a history of amenorrhea

- Are a woman who is trying to conceive

There is nothing dangerous about intermittent fasting since your body will come to no harm if you do not eat for a while. This is the case if you are well nourished and healthy.

Chapter 12:
The Mediterranean Ketogenic Diet

Nutritionists and doctors have conducted numerous scientific studies over the last decade, which has encouraged them to revise their idea of what a healthy diet is. Studies have helped people learn more about the mechanisms and the causes of cancer, arteriosclerosis and diabetes. It is for this reason that the idea of a healthy food pyramid is now disregarded. Grains, beans, starchy vegetables and bread are no longer used as the basis for any diet.

New scientific data and research prove that healthy fat is of utmost importance in a diet. Nutritionists are now combining these principles with the Mediterranean diet. This diet includes a healthy amount of fresh vegetables and nuts and is called the Ketogenic Mediterranean diet. The traditional Mediterranean diet allows you to consume fruit, vegetables, potatoes and nuts, whole grains and olive oil. You can also consume moderate amounts of lean meat, poultry, fish, eggs, dairy products and moderate quantities of red wine. The emphasis is only placed on the consumption of whole and fresh foods, and to minimize the consumption of processed and packaged food.

In a traditional ketogenic diet, at least fifty percent of your food intake should come from fat like butter, coconut oil, eggs, raw nuts, avocado, poultry, red meats, cheese, fish and shellfish. This diet does not include sugar, whole grains, starchy vegetables, beans and flour. We talked about ketosis in the first few chapters of the book. Ketosis is a metabolic state in which your body will break down the stored fat to produce energy. Your body shifts into this state since there are no carbohydrates that it can use to produce energy. This breakdown will lead to the formation of ketone bodies that are used by your body as energy. For you to reach the state of ketosis, you should only consume fifty grams of carbohydrates a day. This means that you can only consume 200 calories worth of carbohydrates every day. The average American consumes close to 600 calories a day, which cannot lead to fat burning.

The Mediterranean ketogenic diet uses a generous amount of coconut oil, olive oil, avocado oil, green vegetables, salads, moderate red wine, fish as the primary protein, fowl, eggs, lean meat and cheese. If you follow this diet, you must eliminate legumes, whole grains, food containing sugar and flour and starchy vegetables like corn, peas and potatoes. Fruit is a healthy choice for a snack, but it is not included in the list. You must choose the fruit with the least amount of sugar in it. This diet is different from other low-carb and ketogenic diets since it focuses more on fish, olive oil, healthy fat choices and red wine.

Anti-Inflammatory Keto (30% More Effective)

Studies show that the Mediterranean ketogenic diet aids in appetite reduction and weight loss. This evidence also suggests that the ketogenic diet is the most appropriate diet for people who suffer from heart disease, epilepsy and diabetes. There is some evidence that suggests that the ketogenic diet helps to reduce the growth of cancerous cells and reduces the effects of Alzheimer and Parkinson's. Apart from this, the ketogenic diet can help patients with headaches, acne, neurotrauma, sleep disorders, multiple sclerosis and autism. Some studies also show that the Ketogenic Mediterranean diet helps to reduce the glucose levels in the body during fasting periods thereby preventing insulin resistance. There is evidence that proves that this diet will help to decrease the levels of triglycerides, LD cholesterol and total cholesterol in the body.

You should remember that there is no single diet, which is good for a person because everybody is unique. You might have digestive issues, allergies or sensitivities that will require you to follow a different type of diet. People suffering from gall bladder disease cannot follow a high-fat diet. People should, however, strive to consume a diet that is rich in healthy fat; they should consume as much as fifty percent of the calories that they consume. They should also consume a moderate amount of high-quality protein, preferably freshwater fish, and lots of brightly colored and green vegetables. They should avoid the consumption of grains, flour products and starchy vegetables, and should avoid sugar, sweeteners and high fructose corn syrup. This is because the sugar will increase blood sugar levels and lead to insulin resistance. This will increase the probability of developing inflammation, which leads to many degenerative diseases.

In addition to this, several nutritional supplements are anti-inflammatory and aid in controlling blood sugar. These include magnesium, omega-3 fatty acids, chromium, curcumin, lipoic acid, resveratrol and vitamin D. You can also supplement any high-fat diet with some pancreatic or digestive enzymes. You should also consume whole food fiber supplements and ensure that you choose those supplements that do not have any artificial sweeteners or sugar.

You should always ensure that you are informed when you make any decisions about your health.

Chapter 13:
Foods to Eat on IF and Sample Meal Plan

Foods to Eat

As mentioned earlier, there are no restrictions or specifications about how much food or what type of food you must consume when you follow IF, commonly known as Intermittent Fasting. You cannot expect to reap benefits from the diet if you consistently consume junk food. It is important to consume a balanced diet to maintain energy levels, lose weight and stick to the diet. If you want to follow the IF diet, you must consume food that is rich in nutrients like whole grains, fruit, vegetables, beans, nuts, lean proteins, and dairy.

Water

It is important to stay hydrated for multiple reasons, even when you are not eating. The amount of water that a person must drink depends on how active that person is. You must ensure that your urine is always pale yellow. If it is dark yellow, it means that your body is dehydrated. Dehydration can cause fatigue and lightheadedness, and if you consume very little food, you are causing extreme harm to your body.

If you do not want to drink plain water, you can add cucumber slices, lemon juice or mint leaves. This can be our little secret.

Avocado

You may wonder why you should consume avocado, a high-calorie fruit, when you are trying to lose weight. The monosaturated fat in the fruit is satiating. A study showed that it is best to consume at least half an avocado for lunch since it can keep you full for longer than if you did not consume the fruit at all.

Fish

The dietary guidelines suggest that one should consume at least eight ounces of fish every week. Fish is not only rich in protein and healthy fats but is also rich in vitamin D. If you do not consume too much food during the day, It is always a good idea to include fish in the meal since it provides enough nutrition. A lower caloric intake can affect your lucidity and cognition. It is best to include fish in your diet since it is considered brain food.

Cruciferous Vegetables

Cruciferous vegetables like Brussel sprouts, cauliflowers and broccoli are rich in fiber. When you consume food at erratic times, you must include food that is rich in fiber to improve bowel movements and prevent constipation. Fiber also helps to keep you full for a long period of time. Therefore, it is important that you consume a lot of fiber when you know you cannot eat for another 16 hours.

Potatoes

It is important to remember that not all white foods are bad for your health. Studies have concluded that potatoes are one of the most satiating foods on the planet and regular consumption of potatoes can help with weight loss. Potato chips and fries do not count.

Beans and Legumes

Beans and legumes are rich in carbohydrates that are required by the body to produce energy when you perform exercise. You should not load up on carbohydrates, but it would not hurt to add some low-calorie carbohydrates in your diet. Foods like black beans, lentils, peas and chickpeas are known to decrease body weight without restricting your caloric intake.

Probiotics

The villi in your intestines love diversity and consistency. The villi need enough nutrition, and they find it hard to survive when your body is starving or hungry, which can lead to issues like constipation. To counteract these side effects, it is important to include food that is rich in probiotics like kombucha, kraut and kefir in your diet.

Berries

Berries are often added to smoothies and are rich in vital nutrients. Strawberries are rich in vitamin C, and it is recommended that you consume one cup of strawberries at least once a week. A recent study concluded that people who consumed strawberries and blueberries regularly had a small increase in their BMI Body Mass Index over fourteen years when compared to those who did not consume berries.

Eggs

A large egg contains six grams of protein and can be cooked in a few minutes. It is important to consume as much protein as possible to build and repair muscles and tissues. A study found that people who consumed an egg instead of a bagel for breakfast ate less throughout the day and were often not as hungry.

Nuts

Nuts may be higher in calories when compared to junk food, but unlike junk food, nuts are rich in good fats. Studies have concluded that the polyunsaturated fat in walnuts can alter the physiological markers for satiety and hunger. If you are worried about your caloric intake, don't be. A study conducted in 2012 found that an ounce of almonds has 25 percent fewer calories than the number listed on the label. When you chew the almond, your teeth are unable to break the almond down completely. There is a small portion of the nut that remains intact in your body which is unabsorbed in the process of digestion.

Whole Grains

When you are on a diet, you are constantly worried about your intake of carbohydrates. You should not be worried about consuming whole grains since they are rich in protein and fiber. It is important that you consume a portion of whole grains regularly since they can boost your metabolism. Go out of your comfort zone and consume grains like bulgur, farro, kamut, freekeh, sorghum, millet, amaranth and spelt.

Sample Plan

This plan uses the 16/8 intermittent fasting pattern. If you are a beginner, you can use this meal plan to help you consume the right food at the right time. This plan will tell you what you should eat or drink and when. The plan is not detailed, and it gives you a range of options to choose from. You must ensure that you always cook your food using healthy oils and fats.

Drink (8 AM – 12 PM)

You must ensure that you drink a lot of liquid before you start to eat. If your workout in the morning, you should drink some herbal tea or a bottle of water fifteen minutes before your workout. You can also drink black coffee since it is a pre-workout booster. You should not drink too much black coffee, though. Read the last chapter to understand why.

Meal 1 (12 PM)

You should consume two eggs, either baked in coconut oil or boiled in water. Consume a bowl of spinach or any other green vegetable and a handful of mixed nuts or almonds. You should also drink two glasses of water, lime juice or herbal tea.

Meal 2 (3 PM)

You can consume 2 cups of quinoa or two sweet potatoes with 200 grams of tuna, beef or chicken. Top the potatoes with a handful of mixed nuts and green vegetables. You should drink two glasses of water with ginger and turmeric.

Meal 3 (6 PM)

You can consume 2 cups of quinoa or two sweet potatoes with 200 grams of tuna, beef or chicken. Top the potatoes with a handful of mixed nuts and green vegetables. You should drink two glasses of water with ginger and turmeric.

Meal 4 (7:45 PM)

Consume a bowl of mixed berries with one apple. Top this with sunflower seeds and cinnamon.

You can follow this sample plan for four weeks and see if it helps you. You can use this plan as a test to understand how your body responds to a change in your eating pattern. Remember that this plan is not exhaustive, and you can always shorten you're eating period. You can gradually increase the fasting period to twenty-four hours and fast for an entire day once your body is used to the intermittent fasting diet.

Chapter 14:
Fourteen: Common Mistakes

The tricky part about intermittent fasting is that there are numerous ways to do it. Generally, over time you will limit the eating window and increase the fasting window. Most people follow the 16/8 intermittent fasting pattern where they do not consume any food for sixteen hours and eat for eight hours. The different methods were covered extensively in chapter eleven. The type of intermittent fasting pattern you choose is dependent on the pattern you are comfortable with and following what best fits your lifestyle.

Since the pattern is a restrictive style of eating, you must ensure that it is safe for you to follow. If you have had eating disorders in the past, you should avoid following this diet.

Some people run into difficulties when they begin the intermittent fasting diet. They often run into those difficulties since they adopt an incorrect dietary approach. If you do choose to try intermittent fasting, you should maximize the benefits. This chapter covers some of the common mistakes that rookies make when they start the diet and helps you understand how you can avoid making those mistakes.

You Are Jumping Too Fast into Intermittent Fasting

One of the main reasons that most diets fail is that they expect you to follow a different lifestyle and steer away from your natural way of eating. This thought makes it hard for one to stick to the diet. If you are new to the intermittent fasting diet, you should never throw yourself into the twenty-four hour fast, because you will feel like hell after the fasting period. If you do want to start fasting, you should have smaller fasting periods. You can choose to fast for twelve hours and eat for twelve hours for a week, and gradually increase the fasting period. You are probably doing this already, so maybe this is the right option for you.

Binging on Junk Food

Most people are under the impression that intermittent fasting is one way to solve every health issue that they may have. It is true that intermittent fasting does help to improve your health and achieving weight loss goals. If you binge on processed food and sugar, though, this dietary regime is not going to do you any good. You must consume whole foods when you follow the intermittent fasting diet. When your body is in the fasting state, it burns the stored fat and damaged cells to produce energy, thereby helping to clean and heal the body. This implies that your body is going to be sensitive to the food you eat. If you do not nourish the body with the right nutrients, you will be hungry all the time. If you want to keep your hunger at bay, you must only consume healthy meals when you break your fast.

Restricting Calories

One of the main reasons people struggle with intermittent fasting is because they control their caloric intake during the eating period. You must learn to listen to your body and always eat until you feel full. The human body is an efficient machine and knows exactly what it needs. You should not restrict your caloric intake and consume food that is rich in fiber and fats. If you do not consume enough calories, you may starve your body.

Not Eating Enough

Some people never undo what they have done when they have fasted for hours because they worry that they will eat too much during the eating period. They believe it will be harder for them to fast during the next fasting period. If you consume fewer calories than required, you are making a huge mistake since your body will be starving. This will slow your metabolism and make it harder for you to shed fat. Regardless of whether you are restricting the quantity of food that you are eating; your body will need an enough food to ensure that the organs function. If your body is starving, you cannot function well and will not be able to think straight. If you feel weak and irritable or are finding it hard to focus, it means that you are not consuming the right number of calories. Here, you should use a food-tracking app to help you count your calories. If you want to learn more about the number of calories you need to function, you should meet a dietician or nutritionist.

Consuming the Wrong Food

When you do not eat often, you should be aware of what food you are putting into your mouth. A diet is not only about the calories, but also about the quality of food that you eat. You should always focus on your nutrition and consume food that is rich in the necessary minerals and vitamins. 500 calories of fried chips and 500 calories of avocados will digest differently and have a different effect on your metabolism and body.

You should always focus on striking a healthy balance when it comes to the macronutrients and fiber. You need to know how much to consume to ensure that your body is healthy. Experts suggest that you load half your plate with vegetables, a quarter of the plate with any lean protein (such as turkey, chicken or fish), and a quarter with healthy starch like quinoa, sweet potato, or brown rice. Since you will be eating fewer calories, ensure that the calories that you consume are nutritious and serve your body well. You should ensure that you do not consume calories from sub-par sources just because you need to consume fewer calories.

Training Harder and Eating Less

If you are not an active person and have never tried the intermittent fasting diet, you should try not to combine the two when you start dieting. You must ensure that you do not take up too much exercise when you have just started intermittent fasting. You must ease your body into fasting and train gradually. Ensure that you do not train your body too much and eat too little because this could lead to severe damage to your health. The human body does need exercise to function efficiently. You must ensure that you do not perform too much exercise since that can damage your health.

Obsessing Over the Schedule

When you follow the intermittent fasting dietary regime, you will understand your body better. You will notice the difference between hunger and cravings. You will also understand whether you are hungry since you are bored, under duress or other factors. You must remember to eat whenever you are hungry and not worry too much about the time. You can break your fast early if you want to eat. You must learn to listen to your body and understand what it needs. It is all right if you were unable to fast for 16 hours. You must ensure that you do not constantly deviate from your schedule.

Not Hydrating Enough

Most amateurs do not drink enough water. You must remember that your body needs to be hydrated to keep the hunger at bay. Water also helps remove the toxins found in your body. You must ensure that you drink at least eight glasses of water a day.

Taking it too Far

You must remember that intermittent fasting is not the best solution for everyone to maintain metabolic health, weight loss, or for increasing longevity. If you have tried the pattern and felt miserable after it, you should re-evaluate if this eating plan is right for you. Some people will tell you that your body can starve for hours and days since our ancestors' bodies did too. What they forget to mention is that this happened tens of thousands of years ago when food was not readily available. This does not mean that this is the right option for you.

Everybody is not built to sustain intermittent fasting. Traditional schools of medicine and health like Ayurveda define people differently based on their experiences with fasting. For instance, Ayurveda has divided people into three types Kapha, Vata and Pitta. The first type of person has extra fat in his body, slow metabolism and is never hungry in the mornings. This person can follow the intermittent fasting pattern with ease. The second type of individual has a varying appetite, can only handle fasting at times and will be thrown out of balance if he or she makes fasting a regular thing. The last type of individual has a strong appetite and cannot stick to intermittent fasting. If he or she does choose to fast, his or her body will be imbalanced, and this could lead to numerous issues.

If you find that intermittent fasting feels like a strain on your body and mind, you should ask yourself this question: is the eating pattern worth the change in the quality of my life?

Chapter 15:
Tips and Tricks

Some of the tips in the chapter are evident, but it is difficult to stick to the diet for most people. When you keep this in mind, you will be able to stick to the diet. The tips mentioned in this chapter will help you stick to the intermittent fasting with ease.

Start Small
Intermittent fasting is not a diet, but a habit. It takes time for a habit to integrate into your life. It is for this reason that you must start slowly because your body will need time to adapt to the new style. It takes at least two months to develop a habit before it becomes an involuntary action. Additionally, if you fail to stick to the diet at times, it does not mean that you cannot develop the habit. It only means that it may take you longer to develop it as a habit.

Always Train in a Fastened State
It is always a good idea to train when the fasting period has ended since the blood sugar levels are at their lowest. This helps to burn stored fat, thereby helping you lose weight. When you perform the

exercise in the fastened state, your body will learn to deal better with glucose.

Find a Friend
When you have someone to help you while you fast and to hold you accountable, you will make more of an effort to stick to the challenge. You can establish an arrangement that works best for both of you.

Always Prepare your Meals in Advance
It is recommended that you prepare your first meal in advance and devour it when you end your fast. If the food is not ready, you might eat readily available junk food instead.

Keep Yourself Busy
You must keep yourself busy when you are fasting. If you do not have much to do, you might constantly check the clock while you wait for the fasting period to end. Alternatively, you can leave your body in the fasting state when you sleep.

Think about Food
It is all right to think about what you are going to eat when the fasting period is over. You do not have to suppress your urges since you are going to think about food constantly. You can look forward to the lovely meals you will consume immediately after the fasting period.

Stay Hydrated

As mentioned earlier, it is important to keep yourself hydrated. If you are bored of plain water, you can add some mint leaves or lemon juice to it. Ensure that you do not add sugar since it could negate the effects of fasting.

Stop Looking at Results Each Day

You must never look for results every single day. You must remember that weight loss is a long process. Instead, count every day when you have stuck to your schedule as a victory since that will bring you one step closer to achieving your goal.

Be Smart and Sensible

It is important that you pay attention to your body. Remember that it takes time for the body to adapt to intermittent fasting. If your body was okay with you fasting for twelve hours today, add an extra hour tomorrow and see what happens. You must learn your limits, but never make it too easy for yourself, or you will end up exactly where you started.

Motivate Yourself

You should ensure that every fast does not end in a feast. You must remember that fasting is about teaching and training your body to become efficient and use what you eat wisely. You must reward yourself with some good food. Never fast only for that reward since the result would then become the reward. You can pat yourself on the back or consume a big meal on a day when you do not fast, but never because you feel like it. This will create a positive association between your mind and the diet.

Some Additional Tips

In this section, we will look at how you can make it easier on yourself when you begin the intermittent fasting eating pattern. It is daunting when you begin the intermittent fasting diet. Some people may experiment with the diet for three days and may not be hungry on the second day of their diet because they have done everything correctly. Instead of motivating yourself, you might tell yourself that you are going to fail because you are already hungry two hours after you broke your fast. There may be days when your hunger pangs were so strong that you could not make it through the fasting period. Some experts may tell you to switch to a high-fat diet, but it takes weeks for your body to adapt to such a diet and you cannot wait that long. Some people choose to back out even before they begin the diet because they are worried that they cannot see it through. What if there was a way to stay calm and confident when you start the diet?

Let us look at how you can do this. Instead of viewing the diet as another difficult path you owe to your health, perceive it as a self-experiment.

- Break the diet down into small and easy steps that will guarantee that you make it to the end of the diet

- Observe your body and analyze your findings

- Establish whether fasting is good for your body

In this instance, you are not committing to the diet, but are trying to learn more about it since people learn by doing. It does sound easier now.

Consult Your Doctor

As mentioned earlier, it is important to consult your doctor before you begin the diet. If you have a medical condition, you must create a plan that does not harm you further. If you feel sick or tired, you must stop the diet immediately.

Keep It Simple

When you are fasting, you must only consume plain water (with lemon juice or mint leaves if desired), black coffee or unsweetened tea. You must keep it this simple.

Keep It Easy

Eat the usual meals during the eating window. Experts suggest that you combine a low-carb and high-fat diet with intermittent fasting to reap benefits. You are only trying to finish the fast. When you decide the fast is good for you, you can look at combinations that work best for your body.

Create A Schedule

A schedule will keep your plan simple. You do not have to adhere to the time since your schedule may vary widely.

Days of The Week

It is easier to fast on weekdays than on weekends since the former are more structured and do not have any external factors affecting your fast. This may vary for you. You should look for days where you do not have the time to eat and fast only on those days.

It Is Okay to Slip Up

You must learn to forgive yourself. You can always pick up from where you dropped off and start the first day again. Try to do what is easiest for you to get back on track.

Identify Your Purpose

You must understand why it is important for you to follow the intermittent fasting diet.

Weight Maintenance or Weight Loss

Fasting helps to control the production of hormones like insulin, norepinephrine and HGH, which makes it easier for the body to burn stored fat and produce energy thereby helping you lose or maintain weight.

Avoid Medication and Relieve Symptoms

Fasting helps to reduce the risk of developing diabetes, heart diseases and inflammation.

Prevent Serious Diseases

Studies have shown that fasting protects the body from cancer and Alzheimer's. Some studies have also shown that fasting helps you live longer.

You must think about your reasons for starting the diet on days when you feel deprived.

Address Your Worries
What is it about intermittent fasting that makes you nervous and want to stop following the diet?

You Can Skip Breakfast
Breakfast is not the most important meal of the day. The reality is that you do not gain weight when you skip breakfast, and it does not help to kickstart your metabolism.

Avoid Snacks
Snacking, like breakfast, does not boost your metabolism and does not help you lose weight. Studies have shown that snacking leads to obesity and liver diseases.

Metabolism Does Not Slow Down
Fasting increases your metabolism and helps you retain muscle while you lose weight.

You should not be apprehensive about fasting because it is not hazardous to your health.

Learn to Be Patient

Again, with the patience theme, you need to be patient with sugar cravings. Cravings only tend to last an hour or so, and no matter how intense they come on, it's important to remember that they will subside! Give yourself an hour, distract yourself by going for a walk, or calling a friend and you may be surprised to see this craving dissipate.

Making Healthier Alternatives

When you're just starting out, it may be hard to kick these cravings overnight, and that's ok. Create healthy alternatives such as the recipes featured in the dessert section of this book. Choose rich foods like avocado to make an avocado pudding instead of indulging in ice cream. Swap in healthier alternative and soon your brain will be wired to crave the healthier version.

Eating Frequently

One of the biggest tricks to keeping sugar cravings at bay is to eat regularly. You want to eat small but frequent meals to keep your blood sugar levels stabilized. Your body will feel more satisfied, so you won't go into that starvation mode where you want to snack on all the wrong foods.

Whole Foods Are Always Better

Processed foods are full of artificial junk that can cause food cravings and blood sugar imbalances. Remove the processed foods from your diet and eat the real thing! You'll feel more satisfied, and your body will be much more nourished eating this way.

Steer Clear of All Artificial Sweeteners

Even though artificial sweeteners are often seen in fad diets, they aren't recognized by the body, and your body can't differentiate between artificial sugar and regular sugar. This can lead to sugar cravings. Remove these sweeteners altogether.

Supplements

Some supplements can help keep sugar cravings at bay. L-glutamine, omega 3's and green tea extract are a couple of commonly used supplements. Remember always to check with your doctor before starting any new supplements.

Get Sufficient Sleep

Often, sleep can be the reason you crave sweets. A lack of sleep can cause your hormones to be out of whack and can lead to cravings. Be sure to get quality uninterrupted sleep every single night to promote health and prevent cravings.

Exercise A Little

Exercise can help ward off sugar cravings as well. Activity raises your serotonin levels the same way a sugar binge does. By exercising regularly, you can keep your serotonin levels up naturally and fill that void without wanting to reach for junk.

Don't Eat Too Many Carbs

This is more of an obvious one, but one that happens quite frequently when you start eating a ketogenic diet. It occurs more if you don't take the proper steps in determining what your optimal net carb intake is. Once you know that number, it's harder to overeat carbohydrates. Remember to measure the number of ketones in your body, and as a rough estimate, the amount of carbs you can consume is between 20-50 grams per day.

Buy Seasonal Produce

If you are purchasing fruits and vegetables from a farmer or a farmer's market, then the product is bound to be seasonal. If you are picking these up from a supermarket, then you will never learn about seasonal produce. The only indication will be their price. The price of produce at the beginning of their respective season is higher since not much of it is available. Not only are out of season fruits and vegetables expensive, but they also lack in quality as well. Depending on where you reside, make sure that you learn a little about the local produce. Make sure that you are buying seasonal produce whenever possible.

Don't Overeat Protein

Although the ketogenic diet is based on low carb eating too much protein is not good either! When you eat more protein than your body requires, some of those extra amino acids will turn into glucose. This can throw your body out of ketosis, so don't go overdoing your post workout protein shakes! To be sure you aren't overeating in the protein department, try to stick with 0.7-0.9 grams of protein per pound of body weight and go for 0.9 grams of protein per pound if you are incredibly active.

Fats Are Your Friends

This diet is only valid if you eat the proper amount of fat! Don't be afraid of fat, especially healthy sources such as coconut, olive, and grass-fed butter. Your body needs this for energy, now that you are eliminating a vast majority of carbohydrate sources. Don't restrict fats or you will be in for some significant mood swings, you will always feel hungry, and your body will start to break down because it has nothing.

Don't Shop Without A List

Make sure that you have enough storage space for everything that you are planning on buying. Fresh food can be left on the shelf for a while, but most of the foods will need to be refrigerated. You can leave the eggs outside, but meat and fish need to be refrigerated. Always make a shopping list before you go shopping. It helps in buying only those ingredients that you need, instead of picking up random elements. Make a shopping list and stick to it. You can safely stay away from all sorts of junk if you do this. Take a couple of minutes and make a shopping list for yourself. There are mobile applications you can use.

Cheap Cuts of Meats

Following a new diet doesn't have to be an expensive affair. Expensive cuts of meats are certainly delicious, but please don't write off the cheaper cuts. Cuts like oxtail, pork shoulder or brisket are quite tasty when cooked properly, and they are certainly less expensive than regular cuts. Cook them in a pressure cooker or a slow cooker, and after a while, the meat will be falling off the bone. Offal and marrow bones are cheap too and they are full of nutrients. Offal is nutritious, but if you aren't keen on eating liver or any other offal you can always add it to other meats and vegetables while cooking. If you start shopping smartly, you can save a considerable sum of money.

Stay Away from Convenience Foods

Convenience foods are certainly an easy alternative. However, if you want to lose weight without burning a hole in your pocket, then it is better to cook your meals at home. If you manage to do your peal prep over the weekend and make a list of dishes you want to cook during the week, you will have your work cut out for you, and it will certainly make it easier to follow a diet.

If you start following these simple tips while starting your new diet, you will be able to increase your chances of success.

Chapter 16:
Frequently Asked Questions

What is Intermittent Fasting?

As mentioned earlier, intermittent fasting is an eating pattern where you shift between periods of fasting and eating. This is not a diet that tells you what you should and should not eat but instead tells you how long you should avoid eating food. There are different types of patterns that you can choose from depending on what works best for you. These patterns are covered in Chapter Eleven. These patterns allow your body to spend more energy on healing and repair. This is not something that can happen if you are in the satiated state all the time.

Who is Intermittent Fasting For?

There are many benefits to following the intermittent fasting diet. These are covered in Chapter Eleven. If you are serious about improving your health and losing weight without making changes to your diet, you should consider the intermittent fasting eating pattern. Since you do not have to make too many changes to your diet, people prefer to follow the intermittent fasting eating pattern. If you want to burn the extra fat while maintaining your muscle, switch to this pattern. It is safe for everybody to follow and provides numerous benefits. The only thing you need to worry about is committing to the pattern, testing it and confirming whether this is something you can do regularly.

Why is It Effective?

Studies conducted in 2014 showed that intermittent fasting was effective since it had an impact on the adaptive cellular responses. This impact helped to reduce inflammation and oxidative damage, improve cellular production and optimize energy metabolism. This study was conducted in rodents, and it also showed that intermittent fasting helped to protect the animals from cancer, diabetes, neurodegeneration and heart diseases. Some studies conducted on human beings showed that intermittent fasting helped to reduce hypertension, obesity, rheumatoid arthritis and asthma.

The Journal of Nutritional Biochemistry published a study in the year 2005 that revealed that there are two reasons why intermittent fasting is effective – increased cellular stress resistance and reduced oxidative damage. This means that intermittent fasting will help your body deal well with stress and cope with fasting. As mentioned earlier, fasting triggers autophagy, which is the process where cells recycle or break cellular debris and dysfunctional protein. This is analogous to cleaning the house or taking the trash out. You should hope that this process happens in your body frequently. I hope this answer helped you understand how intermittent fasting works inside your body.

Why does Intermittent Fasting Burn Fat?

Chapter eleven covered the numerous benefits of intermittent fasting, and most of these benefits were centered on weight loss. Let us look at some of the other ways in which fasting helps to burn fat in the body:

- Increased levels of glucagon, which is a hormone that burns fat

- Increased number of uncoupling protein-3 mRNA, which is an important compound used to produce energy in a cell

- Increased epinephrine and norepinephrine levels that maximize the breakdown of fat

- Increased secretion of the sensitive lipase hormone

- Increased secretion of the growth hormone which helps to preserve a healthy metabolic rate and muscle mass

The idea behind fasting is that your body will begin to rely on the fat stores. Your body will experience this phenomenon when you exercise consistently. Your body will learn to attack the stored fat to provide the various organs with energy.

How Should I Fast to Lose Weight?

This is the same as what was mentioned earlier. The easiest way to perform intermittent fasting is too fast for twenty-four hours. Most studies have used the alternate day fasting method, where you do not eat on alternate days. You can, however, notice significant results when you fast only once every week. You can finish dinner and then start your fast. If you can make it all the way until dinner the following day, you are golden! You should remember that your body will begin to use the stored fat to produce fuel when you are in the fasted state. Therefore, you can burn more fat instead of sugar. This will become a freeing process.

What Should I Eat During the Eating Period?

One of the most important steps of switching into the intermittent fasting eating pattern is to identify how you can shift back into eating food after the fasting period. When you finish your fast, you should pretend that your fast did not happen. You should not compensate for the fasting period or reward yourself. You should wipe the fact that you were fasting a few minutes ago from your memory and eat the way you would normally eat during the day and ensure that you eat responsibly.

If you end the fast at dinnertime, you should eat dinner. If you choose to end your fast at 4 PM you cannot consume anything but a light snack since you can only consume dinner at 7 PM. You should never consume larger quantities of food than what you would normally eat at that time. You cannot end your fast in a few seconds. Therefore, the best thing to do is pretend that you were not fasting and eat the way you would normally eat at the time. Most people tend to crave healthier foods when they end their fast and choose a healthy snack or a smoothie instead of devouring a large tub of ice cream.

Is Intermittent Fasting Bad for Blood Sugar?

Not everybody has low blood sugar as we are led to believe. It is not a common issue with people. You should, however, check with your doctor if you are unsure. People can maintain their blood sugar levels if they are healthy regardless of whether they are fasting or performing intense exercises.

Studies have examined the effects of a twenty-four hour fast, and it was found that fasting did not lower the blood sugar levels. They found that the blood sugar levels did not dip below the 3.5mmol/Liter mark, which denoted that fasting did not lower the blood sugar levels.

Can I Exercise When I Follow the Intermittent Fasting Pattern?

Experts suggest that you perform different exercises even when you follow the intermittent fasting pattern. It is always good to include a variety of exercises, and both yoga and biking are good examples of exercises that will complement intermittent fasting. You should also go through some resistance training once or twice a week to prevent the loss of muscle. You will notice that your energy levels are lower when you exercise while following the intermittent fasting pattern. This is because your body will tap into the glycogen reserves to produce energy, which leads to fatigue. Exercising for short durations and at a high intensity in the fasted state is something you should explore. This will help you lose fat at a fast pace.

Plan Meals Around Workouts

Experts recommend that you perform cardio on an empty stomach, so it is a good idea to go for a jog early in the morning or book an early spin class if you are fasting. It is, however, important that you consume the right food the previous night.

When you know you are going to exercise the following day, you should always think about what you must eat the previous day. Your meals should depend on the intensity of your workout. For instance, if you decide to go for a run or a spin class the next day, you must replenish the glycogen stores with carbohydrates for dinner, which will help you have enough energy for the workout. When you perform cardio after a meal, your body will not have the power to digest, absorb and assimilate the nutrients since your muscles will demand blood flow. It is important to plan your meals to ensure that you do not damage or harm your body while performing the exercise.

The Workouts You Should Choose

If you do not feel lightheaded when you fast, you can perform any form of exercise without any worry. Many athletes find that they are stronger after they fast for an extended period (16 or 20-hour fast).

People are more focused and lucid after a fast. You will derive more benefits when you fast frequently.

If you follow a diet that is rich in carbohydrates for fuel, you must be careful when you perform intense exercises like CrossFit at the end of the fasting period since you may feel dizzy or nauseous. You feel this way when the glycogen stores have depleted, which often happens at the end of the fasting period. If you perform a less intensive exercise, your body will begin to burn stored fat to produce energy.

When to Stop

As mentioned earlier, it is important to listen to your body when it comes to exercise and too fast. One of the major risks is that you may develop low blood sugar if you do not provide your body with the right nutrition. For someone who is new to performing the exercise while following IF, it is recommended that you perform fewer intensive exercises to prevent the dip in blood sugar levels. If there is a sudden dip in blood sugar levels, there is a possibility that you may faint or feel lightheaded.

This does sound scary. It is for this reason that planning is extremely important. Regardless of how long the fasting period is, an important thing for people to consider is the first meal they will consume at the end of the fasting period and how that meal fits into their exercise schedule. It is important to eat complex carbohydrates, protein, healthy fat and fiber during the eating period. On the days when you exercise, you must include more complex carbohydrates, and consume protein and fat on rest days.

Regardless of how intense your exercise schedule is, listen to your body and plan your meals accordingly.

Why do I Get Hungry during my Fasting Period?

Since you are not eating any food and your stomach is empty, you may experience a small growl occasionally. Additionally, the hungry hormone ghrelin will respond to a lack of food in your stomach. It is because of this hormone that your body will begin to react differently, and it will make your brain think that you are starving. The hunger pangs will disappear once your body adjusts to the fasting period.

Why do I get a Headache when I am Fasting?

You should remember that not everybody gets a headache when they follow the intermittent fasting pattern. A lot of research has been conducted on headaches and Ramadan fasting. Women are more susceptible to headaches when compared to men during the fasting period. This is not because of dehydration and is mostly due to withdrawal symptoms. This is like the headaches that you will experience when you quit smoking or drinking abruptly.

If you experience headaches during the first few days of your fast, it is okay since your body is still getting used to the eating pattern. You can treat your headaches normally when you are not fasting. You must remember to get a lot of fresh air and drink lots of water during the fasting period.

Can I Drink?

You can drink, but you must ensure that there are no calories. This does not mean that you can drink diet soda since it is not okay. You should stick to herbal tea or water. Some people choose to drink black coffee, but I would not advise that. The caffeine will increase the levels of epinephrine in your body, which will aid in fat loss. It is, however, a better idea to not drink coffee since you are better off without it, especially because you will not be consuming much food.

You should focus on drinking herbal teas or water, and avoid milk, sweeteners and sugar. You should understand that this is a day of rest for your body, which means that you cannot consume calories of any kind.

Can I Take My Supplements When I Follow the Intermittent Fasting Pattern?

You can take your multivitamins, but it is always a good idea to give your body a little break. If you are taking multivitamins, probiotics or fish oil, give yourself a break for one day. This will also help to protect your body from developing any sensitivity to these supplements or ingredients.

How Often Should I Do Intermittent Fasting?

The answer to this question depends on the type of method you want to use, and if you choose to fast for twenty-four hours, you should stick to fasting once a week. Some people do choose to fast for forty-eight hours every week and have seen great results, but you should restrict yourself to those hours each week.

Why do I Catch a Cold when I Follow Intermittent Fasting?

When you fast, the blood begins to flow into your adipose tissue. Researchers believe that the blood flows into the adipose tissue to help move the fat into the muscles, so it can be burned as fuel. It is because of this that vasoconstriction will occur in your toes and fingertips to compensate for the blood flow, and it is for this reason that you catch a cold.

Will Intermittent Fasting Slow Down My Metabolism?

Despite all the benefits that we have covered, you might still wonder if the intermittent fasting eating pattern will slow your metabolism or bring it to a halt. You have probably been told to eat a small meal or snack every three hours to avoid putting on weight. This is thankfully untrue. The American Journal of Clinical Nutrition published a study in the year 2000 to understand the impact of fasting on resting energy expenditure. The resting energy expenditure is the amount of energy your body will need to carry out the basic functions when you are resting. The subjects were asked to fast for four days, and to most people's surprise, the subjects saw that their metabolism increased for the first three days. In another study, the subjects were asked to fast on alternate days for twenty-two days. The researchers concluded that there was no decrease in the subjects' metabolic rate. In addition to this, people who were on a resistance exercise program and a low-calorie diet did not see an increase in the metabolic rate, and these subjects were consuming at least 800 calories every day for twelve weeks.

In further studies, it was noticed that there was no change in the metabolic rate even if a person chose to skip breakfast. There was also no difference in the metabolic rate of people who chose to eat only two meals a day when compared to those who ate seven meals a day. In other words, food or lack of food does not have anything to do with your metabolic rate. Your metabolism is tied to your weight and muscle mass. If your lean mass goes up or down, your metabolism will also go up or down. I hope these studies showed you that short-term fasting does provide many benefits, and you do not have to worry about sabotaging your metabolism.

Is Intermittent Fasting Safe for Women?

This is a question that many women ask, and this is one of the most controversial questions surrounding intermittent fasting. People who advise women against intermittent fasting state that some studies show that intermittent fasting affects fertility. While this is true, what people do not realize is that all these studies only use the alternate day fasting method. In this method, women do not eat anything every other day. It is for this reason that their hormones act crazy, leading to fertility issues. A woman can fast for an entire day, and only do that once a week. This is safe, and there are no side effects that have been observed yet.

Some research has been conducted which talks about how short-term fasting affects a woman's menstrual cycle. These studies show that fasts that last for as long as seventy-two hours do not affect the menstrual cycle. Even longer fasts do not have an impact on the menstrual cycle of women who weigh a normal weight. Research shows that longer fasts will affect the menstrual cycle of women who are very lean. There is a lot of research, which shows that women of all shapes and sizes can switch to the intermittent fasting eating pattern if they are healthy. Women should only fast continuously for twenty-four hours, and not for longer than that.

If you are a woman and are unsure of whether you should follow the intermittent fasting diet, you can ease into this eating pattern by only fasting for eight or ten hours at a time. You can then increase the length of your fasting period as you see fit.

Should A Person Suffering from Hypothyroid Switch to Intermittent Fasting?

Every human being will be fine if his or her fast does not last longer than twenty-four hours. This is what you should know about fasting: the circadian rhythm is affected by light and food exposure, and some lifestyle practices will help to enhance the natural circadian rhythms. The following practices will help to enhance your circadian rhythm.

Light Entertainment
You should sleep in a dark room, and always get enough exposure to the sun during the day.

Daytime Feeding
You should always eat during daylight. This is to ensure that the light and food rhythms are synchronized.

Intermittent Fasting
You should always consume food during the daylight hours in your eight-hour eating window. A sixteen-hour fast will lead to lower insulin levels and lower blood sugar. The diurnal rhythm is affected if your body has an intense hormonal response to food.

People Say That Fasting Is Not Good If You Suffer from Adrenal Fatigue. Is It True?
This varies from person to person, but if you have full-blown adrenal fatigue, you should perhaps have a shorter fasting period, and have small quantities of food throughout the day to maintain the blood sugar levels.

Conclusion

The Mediterranean diet includes the consumption of liberal amounts of olive oil, fruits, vegetables, lean proteins (predominantly fish), dairy products, and a little bit of wine! This diet places emphasis on the consumption of whole and fresh foods and the reduction in the consumption of processed foods. A regular ketogenic diet recommends that at least 65-70% of your daily caloric needs must be from healthy fats, about 25% from proteins, and the rest from carbs. The keto diet eliminates the consumption of whole grains, starchy vegetables, and sugar in all forms.

A combination of these two diets is the Ketogenic Mediterranean diet. This diet encourages the consumption of healthy oils, green vegetables, lean meats, lots of fish, poultry, eggs, dairy products, and a moderate amount of red wine! Whole grains, starchy vegetables, and all sugars are excluded from the purview of this diet. It is essentially a high-fat and a low-carb diet.

This diet has plenty of health benefits to offer. Since this diet prescribes the consumption of foods that are rich in healthy fats, there will be an automatic reduction in your appetite and in the number of calories you consume. This in turn will help in weight loss. Also, there will be a reduction in the level of triglycerides in your body and your cholesterol levels will be under control. Not just that, this diet is helpful in controlling the levels of blood sugar and insulin in your body. It also helps in treating several brain disorders like Parkinson's, Alzheimer's, and even autism.

The Keto Mediterranean diet is quite a simple diet to follow and by making a few changes to your regular eating habits, you will be able to reap all the benefits that this diet has to offer.

As you come to the end of this book, we would like to thank you for using it as your source of information and guide for a Ketogenic Mediterranean diet. All the information in this book has been taken from reliable sources and will assist you in your transition towards a healthier diet. As you slowly implement the diet, you will see the difference it makes in your life. Remember to be patient and consistent in order to see real results. If you find this book helpful, please recommend it to your friends or family as well.

If you find this book helpful in anyway a review to support my endeavors is much appreciated.

Christine Moore

www.ingramcontent.com/pod-product-compliance
Lightning Source LLC
Chambersburg PA
CBHW020247030426
42336CB00010B/654